The poor,

misunderstood

calorie

Appetite and energy balance, proper

William Lagakos, Ph.D.

W9-BQV-100

Contents

The poor, misunderstood calorie

Counting calories is an ineffective means to determine energy balance or lose weight. The calories in food are *not the same* as those expended by the body. **The poor, misunderstood calorie** explains the concept of calories in the context of nutrition, obesity, and appetite.

Blaming obesity on "eating more than was expended" is incorrect because whether more was eaten than expended can't be known unless the patient is already obese. If you start a diet and exercise routine, the only way to know if you are "burning less than they ate" is if you lose weight; it doesn't matter how many calories you ate or expended. In fact, if your calculated calorie balance doesn't match your change in weight, it is means the calorie count was wrong. There are no other hypotheses under consideration. Therefore, weight loss advice should not be "eat less than you expend," but should be correctly re-stated as "lose weight." In other words, telling someone to "eat less than they expend" in order to lose weight has no more value than telling them to "lose weight" in order to lose weight.

It doesn't matter if a patient actually eats less or burns more; according to the standard definition, it only matters if body weight is lost. Taken to a ridiculous extreme, if a patient loses 100 pounds of fat[1] via liposuction, then they lost weight and therefore must have eaten less than they burned. This of course is absurd but simply means that "eating less and moving more" is poor advice.

Furthermore, if an obese patient undergoes hormone therapy and gains 10 pounds of muscle while losing 10 pounds of fat, then the standard definition would conclude that this patient failed to lose weight. True, technically, but still incorrect because obesity does not mean excess body weight, per se, it means excess fat accumulation.

Lastly, it is practically impossible to accurately count calories even with the most modern, precise instrumentation. The errors in measuring energy expenditure are considerably greater than those required to result in weight change. Similarly, no matter how many calories you calculated were in a specific food, the actual

---

[1] 100 lbs of fat ≈ 350,000 kilocalories. It would take approximately 6 months of complete starvation to lose 100 pounds of fat.

amount of calories in that food isn't even exactly known. Therefore, even with adequate time, motivation, and resources, it is nearly *impossible* to know how many calories are consumed or expended. The dieter who just wants to lose a few pounds of fat will probably never know exactly how much they are eating or burning. So how do we lose weight?

—WSL

The poor, misunderstood calorie

Chapter 1.
The calorie

A *calorie* can mean a number of things. To simplify, I will divide the different meanings into three categories: **Basic Science**, **Food Science**, and **Nutritional Science**. They differ slightly (unofficially) in how they are interpreted and applied.

Basic Science

Just like 'degrees' [Celsius[2]] are units to measure temperature, and a 'meter' is a unit to measure distance, a 'calorie' is a unit to measure heat. More specifically, one calorie is the amount of heat required to raise the temperature of a litre of water by one degree Celsius (i.e., one calorie is required warm one litre of water from 14.5 to 15.5 degrees Celsius).

---

[2] Anders Celsius (1701-1744), Swedish astronomer

Food Science

To measure the calories in a given food, scientists measure the amount of heat produced by completely incinerating the food via electrocution in a *bomb calorimeter*. A bomb calorimeter is a little airtight oven submerged in a vat of water. Food goes into the oven and is ignited (electrically), and the heat produced from the burning food warms up the water. The rise in water temperature is recorded. This method, although sloppy, is fairly reproducible because the oven always works the same way, with the same efficiency. The only variable is the food. The obvious downside of this method for quantifying calories is that your body, unfortunately, does not work as consistently as the little oven in a bomb calorimeter. Our body burns food more or less efficiently depending on a multitude of variable factors (explained further below). In other words, we may get more or less calories from the same food eaten at different times.

The second downside is that when a food company reports the caloric content of a particular food product, the calories for each individual component in that food are simply added together; they don't measure the calories directly, but rather estimate them from the ingredients list. Thus, errors are introduced. And a lot of errors, even small ones, in the individual components can become large errors in the total food product... and we consume things as total foods (not as the individual components). Real people don't sit at the dinner table and eat 22 grams of protein, 50 grams of carbohydrates, and 20 grams of fat. They eat a cheeseburger. And to complicate things further, 22 grams + 50 grams + 20 grams = 92 grams ($\approx$ 3.3 ounces), but a cheeseburger weighs much more than 3.3 ounces (due to things like water weight and air content).

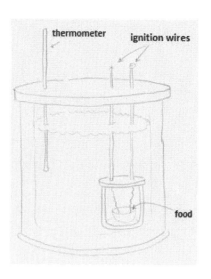

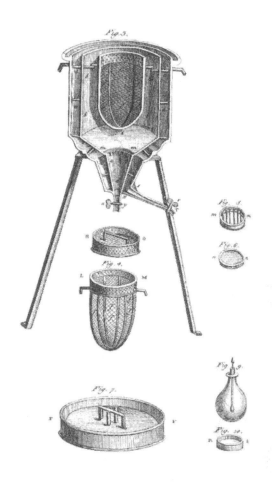

An early calorimeter used by Antoine Lavoisier (1743-1794), the father of modern chemistry. Food would be placed in the center chamber and the outer bath filled with ice. Heat produced from incinerating the food would melt the ice; the more heat produced, the more ice would melt.

Nutritional Science

A *direct calorimeter* is used to measure the calories expended by people. This apparatus is akin to the bomb calorimeter, but much larger and modeled like a small bedroom (as opposed to a little oven). A person stays inside the direct calorimeter for a given amount of time, usually a few hours to a few days, and the amount of heat produced by their body is measured <u>directly</u>. This is the truest technique to measure metabolic rate; there are no formulas or conversions or calculations involved, *it is exact*. Direct calorimetry can be performed with the person running on a treadmill, watching television, or simply sleeping. By analyzing the data from hundreds of people, scientists formulate "prediction equations" which estimate the amount of heat the average person of a particular age, gender, race, etc., produces while running/sitting/sleeping, etc. Although accurate, it only applies to the specific situation that was measured (your metabolic rate while sitting in a bomb calorimeter is not going to be the same as your metabolic rate while sitting at your desk at work)... thus, even when measured with great precision, the information provided by direct calorimetry is limited and not highly applicable to body weight management. Furthermore, your metabolic rate is confounded by factors directly related to being inside of a direct calorimetry chamber, such as when you last ate, whether or not you are nervous or well rested, etc. If a direct calorimeter determined your metabolic rate to be 2,000 kilocalories per day, that may have been true while you were in the direct calorimeter, but it is probably not true all of the time.

Indirect calorimetry is a much less expensive and easier method used to measure energy expenditure. In indirect calorimetry, the oxygen and carbon dioxide in air we breathe and exhale is analyzed. As expected, there is slightly less oxygen and more carbon dioxide in exhaled than inhaled air (...we breathe in oxygen and breathe out carbon dioxide [not exactly, but close enough]). When your energy expenditure goes up, oxygen consumption goes up. Indirect calorimetry *is not* a direct measure of energy expenditure (like direct calorimetry), but is a decent surrogate- we breathe more when we are more active. Importantly, however, indirect calorimetry provides important information about which fuels the body is burning. That is, whether we are burning fat or carbohydrates for energy. The ratio of carbon dioxide exhaled to oxygen consumed, or the 'respiratory quotient (RQ),' is a direct reflection of which fuels are being oxidized. It is not important to understand the biochemistry of this, but in brief: more oxygen is consumed to burn fats, so fat oxidation has a lower RQ than carbohydrate oxidation ($RQ_{fat} \sim 0.7$). Conversely, carbohydrates are more oxidized molecules than fats, therefore less oxygen is required to burn them resulting in a higher RQ ($RQ_{carbohydrates} \sim 1.0$).

RQ: Glucose
$$C_6H_{12}O_6 + 6O_2 \rightarrow 6CO_2 + 6H_2O$$

$$RQ = 6CO_2 / 6O_2 = 1$$

RQ: Fatty acid (oleic acid)
$$C_{18}H_{34}O_2 + 25.5O_2 \rightarrow 18CO_2 + 17H_2O$$

$$RQ = 18CO_2 / 25.5O_2 = 0.71$$

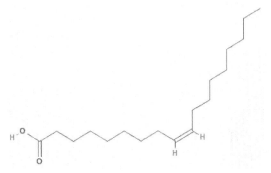

Glucose. Notice the many atoms of oxygen ("O").
All of the corners represent carbon atoms:
6 carbons, 12 hydrogens, 6 oxygens = $C_6H_{12}O_6$

Fatty acid (oleic acid). Notice the relative lack of
oxygen compared to glucose (above).
18 carbons, 34 hydrogens, 2 oxygens = $C_{18}H_{34}O_2$

In an ideal world, we would strive for a low RQ which would mean we were always burning fat. However, respiratory quotient mainly reflects your diet, i.e., a high carb- diet will produce a higher RQ than a low-carb diet. It is also affected by the level of activity: high intensity activities (e.g., sprinting) require higher carbohydrate oxidation, thus increasing the RQ. Low intensity activity burns proportionately more fat. Sleeping, on the other hand, lowers RQ considerably (it is a very *very* low intensity activity).

In sum, direct calorimetry is a proper measurement of energy expenditure via heat production. Indirect calorimetry is a surrogate based on the close relationship between oxygen consumption and energy expenditure.

$$RQ = CO_2 \text{ produced} / O_2 \text{ consumed}$$
$$\text{Fats} \approx 0.7$$
$$\text{Carbs} \approx 1.0$$

Chapter 2.
Why no proper calorie applies to weight loss

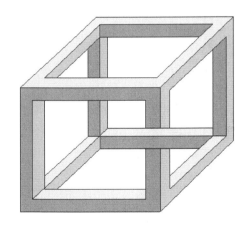

Argument against use of the Basic Scientific calorie: Our body does not use energy to heat one litre of water by one degree centigrade. It uses energy to live, make digestive enzymes in the stomach, synthesize glucose in the liver, climb a set of stairs, sleep, etc. The energy required to do these things, in particular anything related to physical activity, is influenced not only by the absolute amount of work done (e.g., distance traveled), but by the *efficiency of energy utilization* while performing said work. Light bulbs are rated by how much energy they consume, not by how much light they emit. A 100 watt light bulb may emit only 4 watts of light; the bulb is 4% efficient (incandescent light bulbs are notoriously inefficient). A cyclist may use energy at a rate of 480 watts (approximately 413 kilocalories per hour) but the amount transduced to actual forward propulsion may be only 120 watts (103 kilocalories per hour), representing 25% efficiency. The efficiency varies between different activities but can also vary between different people. For an extreme example, think of two people climbing a flight of stairs, with one of them performing a jumping jack on every step. That person will use much more energy to get to the top of the stairs. The distance traveled is the same, but the person doing jumping jacks has a markedly reduced overall efficiency. A more subtle example would be someone whose body is burning more fat to climb the stairs vs. someone burning more carbohydrates. Many factors, including diet, affect the efficiency of energy utilization.

The amount of calories used by our body to do things is variable, unlike the calories required to raise a litre of water by one degree Celsius.

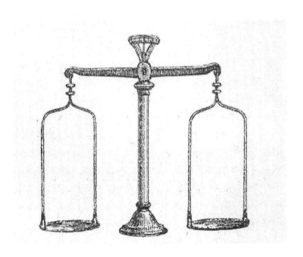

Argument against use of the Food Science calorie: Our body is not a bomb calorimeter. A variety of factors determines how food calories are processed by our body; these factors change over time and are dependent on the sources of the calories, the timing of food intake, and many other things out of our control (the *exact opposite* of the conditions used for bomb calorimetry). For example, 25 grams of protein may yield the same amount of heat (~100 kilocalories) as 25 grams of carbohydrates in a bomb calorimeter; however, 25 grams of protein provides less energy to your body due to things like the *thermic effect of feeding,* which are *not* detected by a bomb calorimeter (more on the thermic effect of feeding in **Chapter 5**).

Another problem is the error involved. Electrocuting a slice of bread may provide, on average, 85-95 kilocalories every time it goes into a bomb calorimeter, but it may provide 75-105 kilocalories to your body. Multiply that by 20 to get your total daily kilocalorie intake and it becomes 1,500-2,100. That is a very large difference. If your doctor or nutritionist estimated that you expend 2,000 kilocalories per day and advised a 500 kilocalorie deficit for weight loss, and you reduced your *apparent* food intake by 500 kilocalories, your *actual* reduction could have been nil (in the case the margin of error is 600 kilocalories).

Argument against use of the Nutritional Science calorie: Although a direct calorimeter is the best way to measure energy expenditure, it is only applicable when you are doing exactly what you did while you were in the direct calorimeter, eating exactly the same thing as when you were in the direct calorimeter, and are the same age & body weight. Even little things like the amount of time sitting in different chairs can affect this. Although individually these factors may not account for much, when added up over the course of a day, a week, or a year, they can account for huge differences.

To say some particular technique is the "best" implies there are numerous others which are adequate and validated. For the purpose of weight management, many will try to calculate their energy balance by adding the calories from food labels and estimating energy expenditure by a prediction equation. This is dreadfully inaccurate.

Rough estimate of energy balance: body weight (lbs) x 10 = daily energy expenditure (kilocalories) = the amount of kilocalories you can eat daily for weight maintenance. This would mean that a 200 lb person expends 2,000 kilocalories and consumes 2,000 kilocalories daily while they are weight stable. Being "weight stable" is defined not by the number of kilocalories consumed and expended, *per se*, but by body weight. Body weight, as measured by a simple bathroom scale, is superior to counting calories to determine energy balance.

N.B[3]. If your body weight is stable over a period of time, then the food calories consumed were equal to energy expenditure during that period. This is true regardless of whether you are lean or obese and is the definition of 'weight-stable' that is used throughout this book.

---

[3] N.B., this is important!

If the abovementioned person consumes 1,900 kilocalories per day for an extended period of time (a 100 kilocalorie deficit), they will lose weight, if it is indeed a true 100 kilocalorie deficit. My contention is that although they may be accurately adding all of the calories from food labels, they may not, in fact, definitively be in negative calorie balance. One clear example of how this happens is that total energy expenditure could easily decline during the dieting period by 100 kilocalories *to match the deficit.* This is not an uncommon effect of dieting. Therefore on pencil and paper, after an extended period of time, the patient should have lost body weight, but the bathroom scale is telling a different story. For the dieter, the best [only] way to determine energy balance accurately is with the bathroom scale. Regardless of any calculations, if the scale says the same thing it did a month earlier, energy balance was neutral during that month. That is a fact, and the only way to accurately know energy balance. Maintaining the same body weight for any extended period of time equates to being in energy balance. This is true regardless of how many calories have been consumed as per food labels, and it is not affected by whichever prediction equation was used to determine total daily energy expenditure.

Furthermore, the amount of food consumed during that period, in calories, was mathematically equivalent to energy expenditure, in calories. You cannot calculate a number for this (by adding the calories from food labels or determining your energy expenditure with a prediction equation) with any helpful degree of accuracy. The best that can be known is that: **if** body weight did not change, **then** the amount of kilocalories you ate equaled your energy expenditure.

As will be detailed in subsequent chapters, food intake is the other half of the equation, and a critical factor in weight loss. If your body weight is reduced over the course of a month, you were in a negative energy balance during that time. Energy expenditure in a given individual at a stable body weight is determined in part by muscle mass, which does not fluctuate widely. Therefore, if body weight was reduced over the course of a month, then food consumption was probably lower (as opposed to experiencing a significant increase in muscle mass to boost energy expenditure). Exercise and physical activity are important for health and wellness, but they do not reliably induce a negative energy balance sufficient for weight loss over the long term... a slightly larger helping of pasta with dinner, an extra scoop of rice, or a couple of cookies easily makes up for the amount of energy burned during an exercise session.

One final point is that the balancing of food intake to energy expenditure is not a conscious act; or, rather, we are unable to actively balance these things in practice. Instead, we eat when we are hungry or at pre-determined mealtimes, and stop eating when we have had enough. If, for example, someone who is in energy balance (i.e., weight-stable) and eating 2,000 kilocalories per day (and by definition expending 2,000 kilocalories per day), then drastically reduces energy expenditure (to 1,700 kilocalories per day, for example, by getting promoted to a desk job or retiring), food intake will eventually decline accordingly. Even though you are eating less than before (1,700 vs. 2,000 kilocalories), you are not in negative energy balance because energy expenditure was similarly reduced. On the other hand, if you are in energy balance (weight-stable) and begin an intense exercise regimen, your food intake will eventually increase to bring you into energy balance. Activity is an important determinant of appetite. This is discussed in detail later on, but in brief, this is why **exercise sans dieting is insufficient to induce long-term weight loss**. Exercise, or "hard work," builds up an appetite.

Chapter 3.
Absolute vs. relative macronutrient abundance

There are many caveats to popular diets. Increase *this*, decrease *that*, watch out for *those*, etc., etc. When trying to understand the principles being exploited by these diets, it is very important to consider what is happening to the nutrients. And here is where it gets tricky. Enter: absolute vs. relative amounts. The 'absolute' amount of a nutrient is expressed as grams per day, for example, "Niko's diet contains 100 grams of protein." The 'relative' amount refers to the percent of total calories derived from that nutrient, like saying "33% of the calories in Jake's diet are derived from protein." When changing the quantities of nutrients in your diet, <u>always consider both the absolute and relative changes.</u>

Some examples of why that is important:

<u>Diets that manipulate carbs</u>

250 grams of carbohydrates (an "absolute" amount) provide approximately 1,000 kilocalories. On a 2,000 kcal diet, 250 grams of carbohydrates equates to a diet that get 50% of its calories from carbohydrates (a "relative" amount). If food intake is lowered by 25% to 1,500 kilocalories, then 250 grams of carbohydrates would then be providing 66% of the total kilocalories; the absolute amount

did not change but the relative amount increased. Carbohydrate consumption would have to be reduced to 188 grams in order to provide 50% of the calories on a 1,500 kilocalorie diet. Reducing carbohydrates to 188 grams on the aforementioned diet is therefore, an 'absolute' but not 'relative' reduction.

Protein (nota bene)

Consider a 2,000 kilocalorie diet that contains 100 grams of protein (100 grams of protein x 4 kcal/g = 400 kilocalories from protein; 400 / 2,000 = 20% protein). A diet that reduces overall portion sizes decreases each macronutrient to a similar extent, resulting in the same relative amounts of each being consumed... that is, fewer grams of protein, for example, but the same *percentage* of total calories derived from protein.

When portions are reduced, the total kilocalorie intake may decrease by 25% to 1,500 and total protein would proportionately decrease by 25% to 75 grams. The relative amount of protein in the diet has stayed the same: 75 grams of protein x 4 kcal/g = 300 kilocalories from protein; 300 / 1,500 = 20% protein (same as before). Some (not me) would say that dietary protein intake has not decreased because it is still providing 20% of the total calories. However, now that this patient is on a weight loss diet, they are likely to be losing some muscle mass. By reducing the absolute amount of protein intake, they will be losing *disproportionately more muscle mass* because of the combined effects of weight loss *and* reduced dietary protein. This is because <u>the *absolute* amount of protein in the diet supports an absolute amount of muscle mass.</u> If you reduce protein intake, muscle tissue is degraded.

For example, a 200 pound woman with 80 pounds of skeletal muscle might be consuming 100 grams of protein every day. This daily intake of 100 grams of protein is contributing to the maintenance of those 80 pounds of muscle. Reducing protein intake below 100 grams per day would result in loss of skeletal muscle, *regardless* of whether she is on a weight loss diet. To some degree this can be compensated by increasing total calorie intake from other nutrients, because protein requirements are determined, in part, by calorie intake. However, increasing total calorie intake to compensate for reduced protein intake would cause an increase in both muscle *and* fat. Not good.

Thus, due to the crucial relationship between dietary protein and muscle mass, protein intake should always be considered on an absolute, not relative, basis.   In other words, *none* of the calorie deficit on a hypocaloric diet should come from protein. With this in mind, the best option for the aforementioned 200 pound woman would be to continue consuming *at least* the same absolute amount of protein per day (100 grams). Yes, this would result in an increased relative protein intake: 100 grams of protein x 4 kcal/g = 400 kilocalories from protein: 400 / 1,500 = 27% protein (compared to 20% protein when the protein intake was reduced in the above example).

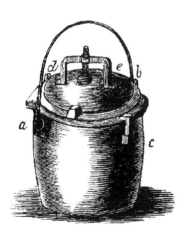

Let's look at some examples

For each of the following examples, the baseline diet (**Figure 1**) contains ~2,000 kilocalories. The first contains 25% fat (59 grams), 25% protein (130 grams), and 50% carbs (260 grams).

	Fat	Protein	Carbs
grams	59	130	260
kcals	527	520	1,040
cal %	25%	25%	50%

Figure 1. Baseline diet: 2,087 kilocalories

_____

_____

_____

_____

_____

_____

_____

_____

_____

_____

Reduced portion sizes

If portion size is reduced by 25% in this example, we get the following:

	Fat	Protein	Carbs
grams	44	98	195
kcals	395	390	780
cal %	25%	25%	50%

Figure 2. 25% reduced: 1,565 kilocalories

Although protein still provides 25% of the calories, total protein intake has decreased from 130 to 98 grams. 98 grams of dietary protein can support less muscle mass than 130 grams. Therefore, muscle tissue will be lost on this diet and metabolic rate will decline[4].

_____
_____
_____
_____
_____
_____
_____
_____

---

[4] Skeletal muscle is a major component of metabolic rate

Reducing only fat

The following diet achieves a similar reduction in calories by selectively lowering fat calories:

	Fat	Protein	Carbs
grams	1	130	260
kcals	9	520	1,040
cal %	1%	33%	66%

Figure 3. 25% reduced calories: 1,569 kcal

This is where we start running into trouble. It is very difficult to achieve a 25% decrease in calories by fat reduction alone. This diet is now deficient in essential fatty acids, and may result in alopecia, poor wound healing, cold intolerance, constant hunger (obsession with food), emotional dysfunction, reduced cognitive ability, etc.

Therefore: Bad idea to lower only fat (**Figure 3**). Bad idea to lower protein [ever] (**Figure 2**). Therefore, by exclusion, it's never a good idea to keep carbohydrates constant when trying to reduce caloric intake. Some of the calorie deficit *must* come from carbohydrates.

_____

_____

_____

Reducing only carbs

The following diet achieves the same 25% reduction in calories by selectively reducing carbs:

	Fat	Protein	Carbs
grams	59	130	130
kcals	527	520	520
cal %	34%	33%	33%

Figure 4. 25% reduced: 1,567 kilocalories

Carbs cut in half; no change in protein and fat. This is the best one so far because protein is not reduced as in **Figure 2**, and it's not deficient in essential fatty acids as in **Figure 3**.

_____

_____

_____

_____

_____

_____

_____

_____

Low-carb, high fat

Although there is technically no calorie restriction on a proper low-carb diet[5], I've reduced the calories in the following example to make it directly comparable the previous examples.

---

[5] On a proper low-carb diet, dieters are only instructed to restrict carbohydrates but not total calories; they are actually encouraged to eat *more* fat to prevent hunger… and yet these diets are successful. However, this is not necessarily a demonstration that 'all calories are not the same,' because it is possible (and likely) that either: 1) food intake is inadvertently reduced; or 2) energy expenditure is increased.

Removing *all* carbohydrates from the diet removes *a lot* of food options; it may be difficult for some people to fully compensate for that deficit by increasing fat consumption. One very important point about this is that on low-fat diets, one *expects* to be hungry because calories are intentionally restricted. On a low-carb diet, since it is not hypocaloric by definition, being hungry is not a necessity. The recommendations of "reduced calories on a low-fat diet" and "no calorie restriction on low-carb diet" are probably how the entire "is a calorie a calorie" debate began.

Low-carb, high fat (continued)

	Fat	Protein	Carbs
grams	87	130	65
kcals	783	520	260
cal %	50%	33%	17%

Figure 5. 25% reduced: 1,563 kilocalories

On this diet the carbs are reduced further, and fat is increased to compensate. Absolute protein intake is not changed and essential fatty acids are not deficient.

_____

_____

_____

_____

_____

_____

_____

_____

_____

Chapter 4.
Buoyant vs. caloric density

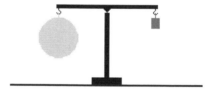

In the image above, two objects are hanging on the ends of a balance. The circular object on the left is obviously much larger than the square object on the right. They are of equal weight; therefore, the object on the right has a much higher density.

A few words on "DENSITY"

The word "density" can actually take on different meanings when used in different contexts. The most common definition refers to the weight of something divided by its volume. A shoe box full of pennies weighs more than a shoe box full of feathers (even though the volume is the same); thus, pennies are denser than feathers.

Buoyant density refers more specifically to how well something floats - If something is denser than water, like a stone, it sinks. On the other hand, if something is less dense than water, like oil, it floats.

Caloric density is the number of calories in a nutrient divided by its weight. It is abbreviated "kcal/g" which stands for kilocalories per gram. One gram of fat provides ~9 kilocalories while a gram of protein or carbohydrates provides ~4 kilocalories. The simplest (though not realistic) example of this would be to consider a meal of 100 grams of a particular nutrient. If it is entirely carbohydrates or protein, it will provide approximately 400 kilocalories (caloric density ≈ 400 kcal / 100 grams ≈ 4 kcal/g). If the meal is entirely fat, it will provide approximately 900 kilocalories (caloric density ≈ 900 kcal / 100 grams

≈ 9 kcal/g). Theoretically, if you were to apply this concept to your diet, eating high fat foods would lead to higher calorie intake, which would promote weight gain. This does not occur, however, because long-term factors such as energy stores and satiety signals have a greater control on food intake than the volume or weight of an ingested meal.

Total calories, caloric density, and appetite

With regard to the intrinsic regulation of food intake, there are two major biological mechanisms.

The first mechanism concerns "fullness," and is regulated by the amount of food in your stomach. Eating a large meal fills your stomach with food, leading to "meal termination," i.e., when you're 'stuffed.' This homeostatic response is good, although it can easily be hijacked. For example, it can be *temporarily* fooled by chugging a lot of water or filling up on fibre. However, excessively filling up like that will lead to at least two distinct compensatory responses. First, you will begin to *eat more*. The body eats for calories; food volume or mass has no caloric value to the body. Second, stomach capacity will begin to increase. This allows for and is often accompanied by progressively *even more food* being consumed before the "meal termination" signal.

The second mechanism relates to energy balance, and is regulated by the energy stored in your body (body fat, adipose, etc.). This mechanism controls "meal initiation," or when you feel hungry and want to eat.

Both meal initiation and meal termination are important to energy balance and the maintenance of a healthy body weight. A low-fat diet is higher in volume and has a lower caloric density than a low-carb diet. Thus, the low-fat diet exploits the "meal termination" scenario. In other words, eating a low fat diet may result in you feeling full sooner because low fat meals take up more volume in your stomach, per calorie, than low carbohydrate high fat meals. This is because: 1) high carbohydrate foods frequently contain a lot of water, which has no caloric value, and 2) carbohydrates are less calorically dense than fats.

Premise of the low-fat diet

The major premise of the low fat diet is that fat contains proportionately more calories per gram than carbohydrates, so eating more dietary fat results in eating more calories, which results in weight gain. Unfortunately, it's not so simple. This volume/calorie disconnect is based on the idea that our brain detects the weight or volume of ingested food, assigns it a caloric value, and relays this information to a long-term appetite regulating system. However, appetite is not the same as fullness. Low calorically-dense foods (high volume; e.g., carb-rich foods) may be more filling *per calorie* but do not attenuate long-term appetite signals as well as calorically dense foods *because of their lower caloric content*. In other words, they might make you full but you will be hungrier sooner.

There are some practical observations that demonstrate why a low caloric density diet should not be expected to be very effective at weight loss.

1) drinking more water with meals enhances fullness but does not cause weight loss. Unfortunately, water does not cure obesity. Water is essential and good-for-you, but it

won't shed the pounds.

2) added dietary fibre enhances fullness but does not cause weight loss. Dietary fibre drastically expands in your gut, which occupies a lot of volume. Again, fibre has a plethora of health benefits, but it will not cure obesity.

The biological regulation of appetite and energy balance is not fooled by filling up on low calorie, high volume (carb-rich) foods, water, or even fibre. In the worst-case backfire scenario, these methods would result in increased stomach capacity, and ultimately bigger portions of food required to achieve "fullness."

<u>examples of caloric density</u>

3 ounces of:

ribeye steak:	174 kilocalories
pasta:	63 kilocalories

500 kilocalories of:

ribeye steak:	8 ounces
pasta:	24 ounces

For 500 kilocalories, you can eat three times more pasta than steak. The pasta will fill your stomach significantly more than the steak. The argument, however, is that you would feel hungrier, sooner after eating a bowl of pasta than after eating a hearty steak. This has been attributed to a variety of reasons. It might be because fewer calories of pasta than steak were consumed, but it might not.

For example,

1. pasta → ↑ glucose and **insulin**
    a. **insulin** → ↓glucose → brain senses low glucose → ↑ hunger
    b. **insulin** → ↑ growth of fat tissue → ↑ food intake to fuel growth

2. steak → fat & protein
    a. fat → signals to brain the presence of an adequate energy
    b. protein → most satiating nutrient

As will be described in detail later, pasta triggers insulin release which lowers glucose and stimulates adipose tissue to accumulate fat mass. Lower glucose could signal 'hunger' to the brain, making you hungry sooner after eating pasta than you would be after eating steak. However, theories like this make sense and are logical, but none have been remotely proven scientifically. So we don't know the mechanisms, but there are plenty of observations.

For example, the low-fat diet was tested empirically in one of the biggest dietary intervention studies of all time. The Women's Health Initiative Dietary Modification Trial included almost 50,000 women and ran for over 7 years (Howard, Manson et al. 2006). The size and duration of this study are enormous. And the design was straightforward: instruct 60% of the women to go about business as usual and instruct the other 40% to adopt a low-fat lifestyle.

At baseline, the women weighed ~77 kg (~170 pounds) and were consuming what is considered an average diet, 39% fat, 45% carbohydrates, 17% protein. During the intervention, the low fat group reduced their fat intake by ~23% and even increased their physical activity by ~14%. The result? 7 long years later?... this turned out to be no better than doing nothing. Nada. No difference between the two groups.

Because the intervention group as a whole ended up right where they started, the researchers were determined to find out why. Therefore they performed a comprehensive set of subgroup analyses to determine who, if anyone, responded favorably to the low fat diet. What did they find? The women in most subgroups were just as overweight as when the study began. However, the subgroup consisting of women in their 50's actually *gained* weight on the low fat diet. Oops. And women who were considered "lean" at baseline (at any age) also gained weight on the low fat diet. Some possible conclusions from this study are: 1) a low fat diet is an ineffective means to lose weight; or 2) if you have a healthy body weight or are middle-aged, a low fat diet may actually cause weight gain. Since energy balance is always maintained, the most likely reason for these findings is that when the women reduced their fat intake, carbohydrate intake increased to compensate. And unfortunately, more women over-compensated than under-compensated. However, the authors concluded that their study *"provides evidence that restricting fat intake does not lead to weight gain."* Perhaps it would be prudent to add "unless you are lean or middle-aged."

Premise of the low-carbohydrate diet

By reducing carbohydrate intake, meals become more energy dense and less voluminous. Eventually, this may lead to a reduction in stomach capacity. In the beginning of a low-carb diet, if the meals are portion controlled, the dieter may not feel sufficiently full with each meal. This is transient because, as stated above, stomach volume is plastic; it will contract to its normal size. Moreover, the higher energy content of the meal will compensate for the reduced "fullness." Theoretically, this higher energy content will also reduce meal "initiations." In other words, you may end up eating fewer meals in a given month, for example.

Much of this has been confirmed in clinical trials. For example, in a study by Stern and colleagues (Stern, Iqbal et al. 2004), subjects were instructed to consume either a low carbohydrate diet with no calorie restriction, or a reduced calorie low fat diet. By the end of one year, the low carb group lost more weight than the low fat group. What was surprising, however (without knowing the results in advance), is that even though the low carb group was instructed not to limit their calories, they spontaneously ate less. If they were eating whenever they were hungry, and this turned out to be less than the low fat group (which it was), than it must be concluded that they were less hungry on the low carbohydrate diet. The energy density of their diet increased markedly but instead of gaining weight, they simply ate less of it. On the other hand, the energy density of the diet decreased on the reduced calorie low fat diet. They were eating a greater volume of food, but this wasn't as satiating as the low carb diet (so they ate more food *and* more calories). These findings refute the premise of a low fat diet with regard to weight loss.

In another year-long study, the low-carb diet was pitted against a low fat diet plus the drug Orlistat (Yancy, Westman et al. 2010). As with the other studies, the low carb group was instructed to eat unlimited calories but very few carbohydrates. In addition to drug therapy, the Orlistat group was instructed to consume a calorie reduced low fat diet. In this study, the low carb group didn't eat less than the low fat group as in the Stern study, but there was one potentially important confounding variable. If a patient taking Orlistat consumes too much dietary fat, they experience steatorrhea[6]. Thus, the Orlistat group had a

---

[6] Fatty diarrhea. Foul-smelling and extremely unpleasant.

superior external motivating factor to reduce their fat intake. In any case, despite eating slightly more calories, the low carb group lost more weight. This doesn't necessarily violate the laws of energy balance because 1) the laws of energy balance are impervious to violation, and 2) energy expenditure was probably higher in the low carb group.

The studies by Stern and Yancy demonstrate an important point. In free-living individuals, a high energy density (low carb) diet does not lead to weight gain. The higher protein and fat content enhance satiety which reduces energy intake. People on a low carb diet do not need to limit their calorie intake because it declines on its own. A calorie reduced low fat (low energy density) diet, on the other hand, has a higher volume which, according to the premise of a low-fat diet, *should* reduce food intake. However, the increased volume alone does not adequately curb appetite. People on these diets must actively monitor their calorie intake (which is dreadfully inaccurate). Furthermore, if a high carbohydrate low fat (low energy density) diet was more satiating, then people would eat less and lose more weight than people on a low carbohydrate high fat (high energy density) diet. But they don't.

Stomach capacity

The size of your stomach, or more specifically, the volume to which it can expand to accommodate a meal, is variable. Consistently eating until you are full will slowly cause stomach expansion, which results in more food required to achieve "fullness." Isocalorically switching to low caloric density foods (low fat, high carbohydrate) entails eating a greater volume of food. The initial weight loss experienced when switching to a low-fat diet is most likely due to increased fullness and earlier meal termination. However, over time, food consumption is increased by additional meals or snacks until stomach capacity increases. This is most clearly exemplified in gastric bypass patients.

Gastric bypass is a procedure which entails creation of a small 1-2 tbsp pouch from the upper stomach, and bypassing the remaining stomach. Stomach capacity is reduced by over 90%. Not surprisingly, however, patients are severely restricted in the amount of food they can eat. Many patients lose a large amount of weight in the months and years following this procedure. Indeed, it is the single most successful treatment for obesity.

One recent study looked into the long-term effects of gastric bypass, or bariatric surgery (Mitchell, Lancaster et al. 2001). This study included 70 patients who had undergone gastric bypass surgery at some point between 10 and 15 years prior. To be sure, gastric bypass surgery is quite severe; accordingly, all of the patients lost large amounts of excess body weight. Furthermore, *most* of them were still significantly leaner at follow-up. What is of relevance to our discussion of stomach capacity is the 10% who regained all of their weight, or the 3 who actually weighed *more* than before. These people weighed more than 300 pounds prior to surgery and accordingly ingested an exorbitant amount of food every day. Surgery reduced the amount of food they could consume by over 90% and some lost > 100 pounds. But somehow, the weight was regained and a small portion of the patients went back to eating enormous amounts of food again. It would be physically impossible to fit that amount of food into a post-surgery stomach. The only way this could occur is by a slow, gradual stretching of the stomach. If you argued that this only happened in a few patients and therefore wasn't true for everyone, I would agree but add that while it might not happen to everyone, it might happen to everyone *who tried*.

Shockingly, this has been documented to occur on significantly shorter timescales (Kolotkin, Crosby et al. 2009). In a study by Kolotkin, a small subset of gastric bypass patients managed to regain almost all, or even more, of their weight back *within 2 years*. In agreement with the 10 – 15 year follow-up study by Mitchell, the subgroup was small. But the fact that it was happened again (independently) confirmed that it is not an isolated phenomenon. Given the severity of the procedure and the physical discomfort associated with overeating after gastric bypass surgery, the frequency of complete weight regain is expected to be low, and that is precisely what is observed.

Disclaimer: Gastric bypass surgery is the single most effective treatment for obesity. In this book, however, these selected gastric bypass studies are discussed in order to demonstrate a concept, the stomach's capacity for expansion, not as a recommendation.

Reducing carbohydrate intake and increasing fat intake will, by definition, decrease the volume of food eaten. As demonstrated by the patients who regained their weight after gastric bypass surgery, food intake is regulated by calories. Gastric bypass can attribute its success in *most* patients to its extreme severity (i.e., for those of whom the discomfort associated with over-eating sufficiently deters over-eating). If surgery is not an option, however, satiety is the only viable target. Dietary fat and protein intake enhance satiety and reduce hunger. Moreover, and as discussed in detail below, it is much more difficult to chronically over eat a diet of high fat and protein compared to a diet of high carbohydrates. The high carbohydrate diet may be more filling, but the stomach can be very accommodating.

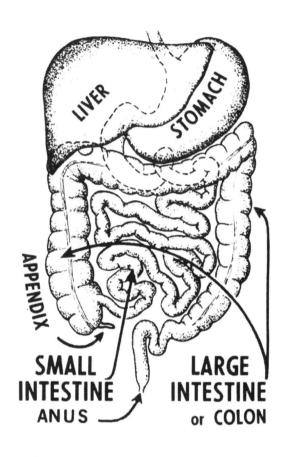

LIVER

STOMACH

APPENDIX

SMALL
INTESTINE

ANUS

LARGE
INTESTINE
or COLON

Chapter 5.
"Is a calorie a calorie?"
-Biochemistry

Is a calorie a calorie? *That* is the question. To make a long story short, this question is really asking whether calories from carbohydrates have the same effect on energy balance as calories from protein or fat. In other words, is it possible to lose more weight on an isocaloric low-carb or low fat diet? It seems simple and straightforward, but is actually a rather difficult question to address from a biochemical *and* practical standpoint.

The paradox:

-to lose weight, you must "eat less" (consume fewer calories than you are expending)
[suggests a calorie is a calorie]

- but people lose more weight on a low-carb diet with no calorie restriction than on a reduced calorie low fat diet
[suggests a calorie is not a calorie]

The questions:

-are low carbohydrate diets more effective because they inevitably result in calorie reduction? (even though calories are technically not restricted)
[suggests a calorie is a calorie]

-do low carbohydrate diets induce a 'metabolic advantage' whereby fat is preferentially burned instead of stored, causing 'nutrient partitioning?' ...
[suggests a calorie is not a calorie]

-does said 'nutrient partitioning' expend energy and therefore promote a negative energy balance?
[suggests a calorie is a calorie]

Another way to break it down: take two people, Paige and Lola. Both have a baseline energy expenditure of 2,050 kilocalories per day and are weight stable. Paige decides to try the traditional reduced calorie low fat high carbohydrate diet. Lola tries the high fat high protein low carb diet. [generally, calories are not restricted on a low carb diet, but in order to address this question directly, we'll say that both girls reduced calorie intake to the same extent]

Who loses more weight?

1. If a calorie is a calorie, then theoretically both girls lose the same amount of weight.

2. If there is some sort of metabolic advantage to low-carbohydrate diets, then Lola loses more weight and we conclude that all calories are not created equal.

This is where current technology becomes the limiting factor. Technically, there are more possibilities. What if one of the diets alters energy expenditure?

3. If Lola loses more weight than Paige, then we would conclude a calorie is not a calorie... BUT what if she lost more weight because the diet increased her energy expenditure? Does that mean that we weren't properly addressing the calorie debate?

See? It is complicated. In the above example, energy expenditure would need to be measured *continuously*, in a direct calorimeter. And even in the most extreme cases, the differences are expected to be very small, so the statistical power to detect a difference would require a lot of subjects studied for a long duration. These experiments are impractical, inconvenient, and expensive.

The following are some of examples of which calories are calories, and which are not :/

1. Protein

More energy is required to digest and assimilate dietary protein than carbohydrates. In other words, eating an additional 100 kilocalories of protein will cause a smaller energy surplus than eating an additional 100 kilocalories of carbohydrates. Conversely, reducing carbohydrate intake by 100 kilocalories causes a relatively greater energy deficit than reducing protein intake by 100 kilocalories (with protein, some of the calorie deficit would be offset by the energy saved by *not* digesting and assimilating the protein). The nutrients may produce the same amount of heat in a bomb calorimeter, but they do not provide the same amount of energy to the body...

don't eat less protein

2. Carbohydrates

Glycemic index and glycemic load are measurements of how much certain foods affect blood glucose. White bread causes a greater increase in blood glucose than, for example, whole grain pasta, and therefore is assigned a higher glycemic index value (see figure below). In terms of energy balance, however, glycemic index does not matter. Low glycemic index diets may reduce disease burden but have failed to produce significantly greater weight loss than high glycemic index diets. In other words, calories from high glycemic index carbohydrates *are the same as* calories from low glycemic index carbohydrates. Eating large amounts of high-fructose corn syrup is certainly bad for you, but in terms of weight loss, this would suggest they may not be much worse for energy balance per se than eating an isocaloric big bowl of rice.

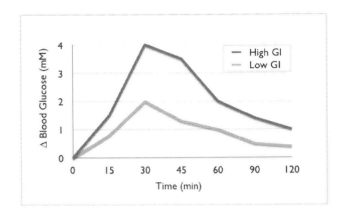

Figure 1. Blood glucose excursions after consuming a high or low glycemic index test meal.

Gluconeogenesis

Essentially, there are two conditions naturally associated with carbohydrate restriction.

1) During a low carbohydrate diet, carbs are intentionally restricted to very low levels

2) When fasting, all nutrients (including carbohydrates) are restricted. Broadly, this refers to starvation, but also applies to sleeping.

When carbohydrates are restricted, the brain still has a mandatory fuel requirement. Most of the time, this is met by glucose. After a meal, dietary carbohydrates are the primary source of glucose for the brain. Dietary protein is another source, as will be discussed below. When fasting, on the other hand, the body makes glucose through a process known as 'gluconeogenesis.'

Gluconeogenesis occurs primarily in the liver and is an expensive process; the liver requires energy input to synthesize glucose. Energy input comes from fat oxidation. So when glucose is coming from gluconeogenesis, there is a negative fat balance relative to when it is coming directly from the diet. Thus, on an *isocaloric* low carbohydrate diet, energy expenditure is increased due to gluconeogenesis. This is an important point in the calorie debate: the foods you eat can raise or lower energy expenditure.

The major precursors for gluconeogenesis are amino acids (from protein), glycerol (from triacylglycerols [fat]), or lactate. Skeletal muscle or dietary protein is degraded to provide the amino acids for gluconeogenesis. Adipose tissue or diet provides the glycerol and fat to fuel gluconeogenesis. When this is increased, as during fasting or low carb diets, the fats are generally only partially oxidized creating 'ketones.' Ketone levels in the blood and urine increase inducing a state known as 'ketosis.'

Side note on ketosis: ketones contain energy; when they are excreted in the urine this essentially wastes energy, thus promoting a negative energy balance. This is neither measured by a bomb nor a direct calorimeter! Is it a metabolic advantage?

Furthermore, although the added energy required for gluconeogenesis *does* increase energy expenditure and *is* measured by directly calorimetry, does *it* qualify as a metabolic advantage?

Wait a minute, if the amino acids come from skeletal muscle, won't this result in muscle wasting? If you are fasting, then yes. However, low carbohydrate diets are often modestly higher in protein than calorie reduced low fat diets. This reduces the requirement for skeletal muscle amino acids thus preserving lean mass.

People consistently lose more weight on low carbohydrate diets than on low fat diets, although this doesn't prove there was a metabolic advantage *per se*. Does it matter?

A study was done to try and quantify the impact of gluconeogenesis on energy expenditure (Veldhorst, Westerterp-Plantenga et al. 2009). In this study, 10 young healthy men were fed either a mixed diet or one intended to maximize gluconeogenesis. This included high protein (30% vs. 12%) to provide all of the essential gluconeogenic precursors (amino acids), and low carbohydrates (0% vs. 55%) to stimulate the need for gluconeogenesis by reducing the input of dietary glucose.

The investigators wanted to keep carbohydrates low also because carbohydrates stimulate the release of insulin which inhibits 'glucagon,' a pro-gluconeogenic hormone. Insulin also suppresses the release of other precursors for gluconeogenesis such as amino acids from muscle and glycerol from adipose, and inhibits the release of free fatty acids from adipose tissue which are necessary to provide fuel for gluconeogenesis.

So basically, although the two diets contained differing amounts of all the macronutrients, they were designed to test the effects of gluconeogenesis on energy expenditure, not necessarily the effects of different diets on gluconeogenesis. In this regard, the diets were chosen well. Furthermore, the researchers also reduced the subjects' glycogen stores with exhaustive exercise in order to remove all possible hindrances to gluconeogenesis[7].

They found that, indeed, a high protein, zero carbohydrate diet enhanced energy expenditure by approximately 5%. Increased gluconeogenesis accounted for 42% of the increase in energy expenditure. That may not seem like a lot, but 5% of 2,500 kilocalories is 125 kilocalories. An energy surplus of 125 kilocalories per day for a year equates to over 10 pounds of fat mass. Importantly, they found that the energy cost to produce glucose via gluconeogenesis was almost a third of the actual energy content of the product, glucose (like spending $0.33 to earn a buck as opposed to picking one up off the ground). It is a wasteful process. In other words, gluconeogenesis burns calories.

If gluconeogenesis only accounted for 42% of the increased energy expenditure, what accounted for the other 58%? These were not measured, but urea synthesis and increased protein turnover may have accounted for some.

---

[7] Hepatic glycogen is another non-dietary source of glucose

Respiratory quotient was reduced, reflecting greater fat oxidation. This may have been partially due to the fat oxidation requirements of gluconeogenesis, but primarily because the body burns what you give it; increased fat in the diet results in higher fat oxidation.

A disadvantage of this study was that it only lasted 1.5 days. It is not known how these results would differ if the study did in fact last for a year. However, this study is important because it illustrates the fact that diet can alter energy expenditure. Calories from a high protein diet may be worth less than calories from other nutrients because some of that energy is used for gluconeogenesis and protein synthesis, *and is not available for storage*.

Chapter 6.
"Is a calorie a calorie?" -Nutrition

In the real world, energy expenditure is a major determinant of food intake. *(Of course 'availability' is important also; that is, if you are offered a sweet delicious snack one day and not the next day.)* Furthermore, there is a strong correlation between total daily activity level, hunger, and food intake. For example, a bedridden patient experiences less hunger and eats less than an athlete training for a marathon. A child that is growing (another form of energy expenditure that is often overlooked because it is not easily observed in the short-term) will have higher total energy expenditure and therefore eat more than a similarly sized adult who has the same amount of muscle mass. Normalizing food intake to fat-free or muscle mass is important because it is this component (muscle) that expends the most energy. Imagine your leg muscles contracting while you climb a set of stairs. Your leg muscles are burning a lot of calories under these conditions. Adipose tissue (fat mass) never contracts like that under any conditions, not even when fat is being stored at a very high rate. Thus, adipose burns fewer calories than skeletal muscle. Many tissues consume energy, just not as much as skeletal muscle.

Low-fat food choices

You might think that by switching from regular milk to [processed] reduced fat milk, you are tricking your body into losing weight. However, according to 'dietary displacement,' reduced calories from the milk will be compensated by either drinking more low-fat milk or eating more of something else to make up the deficit. Thus, by switching to reduced fat milk, total food intake (by volume) will increase ... and unfortunately this will most likely result in greater consumption of sugars simply because they are the most accessible foods.

The theory to try and match your true daily caloric expenditure with your actual caloric intake is problematic. Not even scientists are *that* good. 1. There is extreme variability in day-to-day energy expenditure and 2. we are unable to accurately recall/determine/measure food intake.

During weight maintenance, if the dietary macronutrient composition is changed, then energy expenditure changes (independent of changes in easily observable things like physical activity). This is magnified during weight loss. Moreover, when there is an active attempt to reduce caloric intake, 'dietary displacement' takes place... this means that on the one hand, certain calories are reduced (usually in the form of fat calories), but they are partially compensated by an increase in other calories (usually sugars, due to their tastiness and accessibility). This is probably subconscious... recall the abovementioned chicken & rice dinner; to compensate for reduced calories, one will increase their intake of rice (this is a relatively OK type of compensation; it can also occur with binges of dessert foods that go unreported). In other words, since food intake is primarily controlled by calories, a conscious attempt to reduce calories (by decreasing fat intake) is usually matched by a subconscious increased intake of other calories (usually sugars).

Appetite and calories

An overweight person and lean person can eat the same amount of fat (on an absolute basis [grams]). The difference may be that the overweight person consumes more carbohydrates (on an absolute basis), resulting in a much greater quantity of food *and* total calories being consumed. In some cases the difference in calories is small but the macronutrient composition of the diet is the culprit, causing excess fat accumulation and ultimately obesity. Even though the total fat content of a low fat diet is much lower than that in a low carb diet, fat storage is more efficient in the former due to high insulin levels. Thus, the concept of calories becomes almost meaningless when we consider things like insulin, adipose tissue dynamics, and fat storage.

Reducing calories by decreasing fat intake does not affect the relationship between calories and satiety; although it may be lower in calories, the low fat (high carbohydrate) meal will be larger, and may fill you up sooner, but that is only half of the equation. The relationship between calories and satiety is distinctly different from the relationship between "fullness," or gastric distension, and satiety. When your brain catches on, you end up eating more, usually in the form of carbohydrates since this is a low fat diet. Reducing carbohydrate intake, on the other hand, will lead to a greater overall reduction in the volume of food eaten, *even in an isocaloric scenario* due to the increased caloric density of low carb high fat foods (e.g., steak vs. pasta). However, calories from dietary fat and protein are better connected with the satiety signal than carbohydrates according to the abovementioned examples of spontaneous reductions in food intake on low carbohydrate diets. Thus, 1.) it is easy to over eat carbohydrates, and 2.) insulin promotes fat storage… which seemingly supports both sides of the calorie debate (the contribution of "overeating" to weight gain supports "a calorie is a calorie;" and the effects of insulin on fat storage suggests some calories are worse than others).

> **it is as easy to**
> *over eat a high carbohydrate diet*
> **as it is to**
> *under eat a low carbohydrate diet*
> **-WSL**

final word on caloric density and food volume

Whereas lowering the fat content of a meal does little to the overall volume, the accompanying increased carbohydrates make the meal significantly larger.

Consider a baked potato with butter. Remove the butter. The volume of the meal has not changed much. To replace those as carbohydrates would almost require another baked potato. Meal volume would be markedly increased.

The opposite is not true, however. Consider the same baked potato with butter. Remove the potato. The volume of the meal has shrunk considerably. To replace those calories as fat would require about half a teaspoon of butter. The size does not change much.

But fat and protein rich foods are more satiating, suggesting calories matter more to satiety than the size of the meal. Drinking more water with your meals increases the volume of the meal, but will not reduce your appetite sufficiently to induce weight loss.

The observation that carbohydrate-rich meals induce less satiety than protein and fat-rich meals is not new, although exactly how it occurs is unknown. When you eat a large meal, nutrients flood into the bloodstream. These nutrients may ultimately signal to the brain that you are well-fed. The role of insulin is to get these nutrients out of the bloodstream as quickly as possible. One possibility is that by clearing out those nutrients so quickly, the carb-induced insulin secretion ultimately *reduces* the fed signal to the brain, causing you to be hungry again. Dietary fat (e.g., eggs, meats, etc.), on the other hand, tends to stay in the bloodstream for longer than carbohydrates.

Water quenches thirst. Food should satisfy hunger. Calories should satisfy hunger, equally, if they are providing the same amount of energy to the body. But calories from fat and protein satiate better than calories from carbohydrates. This logic supports that all calories are not the same, due to their effects on appetite. If the focus were to shift from strictly energy balance to weight loss, this may be the more important interpretation of the energy debate. Combined with the fat-storing effects of insulin, the conclusion must be that all calories are not the same. Biochemists believe obesity is caused by a positive energy balance. Nutritionists believe obesity is caused by excessive fat storage. A suitable compromise might read as follows: carb-rich foods are easily over-eaten, producing a positive energy balance. The accompanying elevations in insulin cause net fat storage. The extent of the positive energy balance necessary is discussed in detail in Chapter 12.

However, a carb-rich diet does not have to be over eaten excessively, or grossly hypercaloric, to induce obesity; quite the opposite in fact. Maybe the "experts" were right all along when they claimed that an excess of only 10 or 20 kcal / day, over the course of years, would result in obesity. They just failed to mention that insulin is required to invest the calorie surplus into fat tissue, which implicates carbohydrates. Maybe all calories are calories, but not all calories are equally obesogenic.

In biochemistry, a calorie is a calorie;

in nutrition, it is not.

Diets that reduce portion size vs. the importance of muscle mass

The weight lost during a diet is usually comprised of 2/3 fat and 1/3 muscle. In other words, if a dieter loses 15 pounds, they probably lost approximately 10 pounds of fat and 5 pounds of muscle. Although this loss of metabolically active muscle is unfortunate, the outcome is still OK. For example, a 200 pound woman with 30% body fat (200 x 30% = 60 pounds of fat mass), after losing 15 pounds would weigh 185 pounds and with 50 pounds of fat mass. She lost 10 pounds of fat and her total body fat was reduced from 30% to 27%.

However, the loss of muscle mass causes the reduced metabolic rate experienced by successful dieters. In addition to the many other negative effects of reduced muscle mass, this also hinders further weight loss. One way to combat this is to increase total (absolute) protein intake. (and yes, this also means that *relative* protein intake will increase.)

Dietary protein requirements are affected primarily by muscle mass but also by total calorie intake. This is true at both extremes: increasing calorie intake reduces dietary protein requirements, and reducing calorie intake increases dietary protein requirements. Therefore, to apply this to the situation of the aforementioned 200 pound woman, her *best* option would be to *increase* total protein intake from, for example 100 grams to 125 grams: 125 grams of protein x 4 kcal/g = 500 kilocalories from protein; 500 kilocalories was 25% on a 2,000 kilocalorie diet and is 33% on a 1,500 kilocalorie diet. Thus the absolute *and* relative amounts of protein in the diet are increased. By doing this, muscle mass is much more likely to be retained. And this is supported by clinical trials; high protein diets consistently result in more successful *long-term* weight loss.

For example, a 2004 study by Astrup and colleagues, was designed to test whether the amount of dietary protein could affect maintenance of a reduced body weight (Due, Toubro et al. 2004). In this study, 40 obese subjects were assigned to either a low protein (15%) or high protein (25%) group. Both groups consumed low fat (30%) so the difference in calories was made up for by carbohydrates. Urinary nitrogen, a marker for dietary protein intake, was markedly increased for the entire 1st year in the high protein group, confirming their adherence to the dietary intervention. As expected, the high protein group lost significantly more weight despite eating slightly more calories per day. What does this say about the satiating effect of increasing dietary protein? The diets were both ad libitum (unrestricted calories). The high protein group lost more weight, and still consumed more calories than the low protein group during the latter half of the study when they were no longer losing weight, but maintaining a reduced body weight.

Perhaps just like how energy expenditure is routinely normalized for fat-free mass, "appetite" should be normalized for energy balance? Or perhaps "appetite" should be normalized to specific foods? That is, you may be hungry for 2,000 kilocalories of food from a low protein diet, or 2,100 kilocalories of food from a high protein diet; both diets will keep you in energy balance. In other words, both diets were ad libitum; **subjects in the high protein group were *hungry for less [energy] than they were expending***, to a greater degree than those in the low protein group. Does this mean the high protein diet was more satiating? Does this depend on energy balance? In other words, if you're hungry for 2,000 kilocalories of diet

A or 2,100 kilocalories of diet B, but you will lose weight on 2,100 kilocalories of diet B because something in diet B elevates your energy expenditure. Does this mean that diet B was more satiating, even though you ate more, because it induced a greater energy deficit? These questions keep me up at night.

Back to the study: the high protein group had higher food intake but lost more weight. This doesn't mean the laws of energy balance were violated. And we somewhat expect the high protein group to exhibit higher energy expenditure for 3 reasons: 1) higher dietary protein should result in a higher thermic effect of feeding; 2) the high protein should have maintained skeletal muscle better than the low protein (skeletal muscle contributes largely to total energy expenditure); gluconeogenesis, urea synthesis, protein turnover, etc. The thermic effect of feeding was not measured, but fortunately body composition was which confirmed that the higher protein diet sustained lean mass to a greater degree than the low protein diet. Moreover, fat mass was significantly lower in those following the high protein diet. In other words, **they got leaner without a more negative energy balance**. In this context, this statement is meant in a relatively abstract way and is very specific to the comparison *between* groups; they lost body weight, so yes, energy expenditure was greater than energy intake; but they were eating more than the low protein group, so relative to the low protein group, energy balance was not negative. Admittedly, this isn't really what is meant by "energy balance," but the point must be made clear: **the high protein group was eating more than the low protein group yet they were losing more fat mass**.

And the most important finding of this study... some more background first. For the first 6 months, subjects received an intensive dietary intervention; all their food was provided. For the next 12 months they were regularly counseled. At the 24 month follow-up, only body weight was reported. So from baseline until 12 months, we know that the high protein group was eating more protein and calories, and losing more fat mass than the low protein group. Dietary information was not recorded after 12 months, and the difference in body weight between the groups decreased, so we can assume their diets drifted back to normal. At 24 months, significantly more people in the high protein group kept off at least 22 pounds compared to the low protein group. More specifically, 20% of subjects in the high protein group were still 22 pounds lighter while 0% of subjects in the low protein group were. Similar results were seen at 12 months. In other words, even when weight loss *does* occur on a low protein diet, it is not very much and it is not sustained. These two things can most likely be directly attributed to the metabolic effects of increased dietary protein.

Furthermore, this study was not cherry-picked simply to prove a point. This was a very powerful study: 50 subjects, all food provided for first 6 months!, intensive dietary counseling, numerous body composition measurements, two-year follow-up!; this was a very expensive and labor-intensive study. As stated in earlier chapters, most food intake measurements are notoriously inaccurate; however, these researchers confirmed their food intake data with biomarkers (dietary protein → urinary nitrogen). Furthermore, the dropout rate was low. This was probably due to the ad libitum feeding regimen; "eat as much as you want" is easy to stick with. In practice, all of the subjects ate less, which people commonly do when they are being watched, but it is still a very lax set of rules to follow.

Conclusion: the recommendation to reduce portion sizes to lose weight has a critical flaw, which is that it treats all calories the same. They are not.

Some thoughts on diet studies

It is extremely difficult to measure food intake accurately. On top of all the problems with measuring calories discussed in the beginning of the book, it is equally as difficult to get accurate food intake data. For example, serving sizes are rarely uniform, it is difficult to gauge food weights, and the water content of foods varies widely. To make matters worse, unhealthy people overestimate their good habits and underestimate their poor habits. Overweight people overestimate their physical activity level and underestimate their body weight and how much they eat.

There are a multitude of techniques to ascertain food intake data in a large population. Whether it is the inexpensive but inaccurate food frequency questionnaires or the expensive yet more accurate food diaries and 24 hour food recalls, each has its own distinct set of strengths and drawbacks. Cost is often limiting. A bigger sample size makes a study more statistically powerful, but then the researcher has to compromise by using a cheaper means to determine food intake. In some cases, the inaccuracies of food frequency questionnaires may average out if the subject population is very large.

In other cases, it is best to trust food diaries or 24 hour recalls.

BUT, the take-home message is that much of what we know about nutrition comes from a mix of those techniques. If someone argues that the results from a diet study are wrong because the food intake data were unreliable, then that person must also admit that much of what they know about nutrition is wrong too because it was most likely learned from similar studies. My opinion is that these methods are not perfect, but they are the best we have.

On the other hand, there are instances when cheap food intake data can be extremely accurate. For example, if a researcher wants to know about meat consumption, they can simply ask how often in the past week or two has the subject eaten meat. There is a big difference between someone who can't remember eating meat in the past two weeks and someone who said 'every day.' Thus, the comparison between these two groups based on "low" and "high" meat consumption is probably accurate. If the subject has a poor memory or it simply slips their mind, even in the worst case scenario, a daily meat eater won't say they haven't had meat for two weeks unless they are intentionally trying to deceive the investigator; usually, there is little motivation to deceive the investigator.

Lastly, biomarkers are superior measurements of food intake. A biomarker is something in blood or urine that can be objectively measured consistently and accurately and is directly related to consumption of a specific food. For example, when someone eats more protein, serum and urinary nitrogen increases. If someone eats very low carbohydrates, serum and urinary ketones increase. Tomatoes and carrots increase the levels of carotenoids in the blood. These things are phenomenally more accurate than food frequency questionnaires, food diaries, and food recalls, but they are very expensive and there are only biomarkers for a few food items. I suspect biomarkers will become the gold standard within the next decade or so.

Lies, damned lies, and statistics

1) it is much less accurate to make comparisons between people with small differences in consumption of a certain food. And you absolutely must confirm the actual size of the changes, not just whether or not they are statistically significant. For example, if researchers discovered, after following 10,000 subjects for 10 years, that there is a 99.99999% chance that eating stones for breakfast will increase your lifespan, I would believe that eating stones for breakfast would increase my lifespan and it would also be front page news. But sifting through the data, you might find out that it only increases your lifespan by 4 minutes. Would you still eat stones for breakfast? This is just one of the ways in which data presentation can be deceiving.

2) another example: factor X doubles your chances of dying. That sounds big, right? But what if your chances of dying are one in a million to begin with. Enter factor X and now your chances of dying are 2 in a million. Going from one in a million to 2 in a million is doubling, technically, but the researchers don't always mention the millions.

Normal incidence rate:
    1/1,000,000 = 0.0001%

After exposure to factor X:
    2/1,000,000 = 0.0002%

Increase in relative risk:
        (0.002% - 0.001%)/0.001% = 100%
        A 100% increase is equal to a doubling.

Increase in absolute risk:
        0.002% - 0.001% = 0.001%

The relative risk doubled but the absolute risk only
increased by 0.001%.

3) Lastly, studies like Framingham, DART, GSSI,
    Ni-Hon-San, etc., were thorough in their food
    intake measurements, followed large
    populations for long periods of time, and
    reported data in a straightforward manner; the
    results from such studies have considerably
    more gravitas.

Chapter 7.
the good, the bad, and the not-so-bad after-all

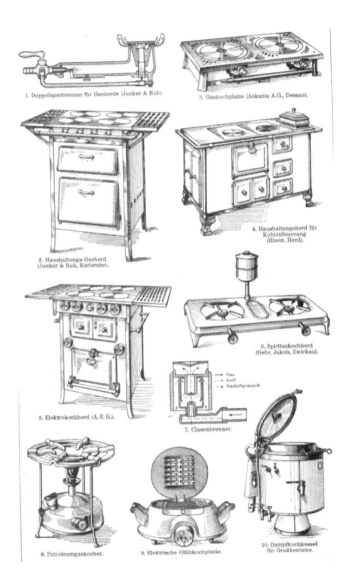

1. Doppelsparbrenner für Gasherde (Junker & Ruh).

2. Gaskochplatte (Askania A.G., Dessau).

3. Haushaltungs-Gasherd (Junker & Ruh, Karlsruhe).

4. Haushaltungsherd für Kohlenfeuerang (Rhein. Herd).

5. Elektrokochherd (A. E. G.).

6. Spirituskochherd (Gebr. Jakob, Zwickau).

7. Clasenbrenner.

8. Petroleumgaskocher.

9. Elektrische Glühkochplatte.

10. Dampfkochkessel für Großbetriebe.

Dietary protein

Dietary protein is essential. It one of the most important, if not *the* most important macronutrient required for optimal health. Everybody's protein requirement is different, but a rough gauge is take your body weight in pounds and divide it by two. This will give you an estimate of the amount of protein you should be eating per day in grams. For example, a 150 pound woman should be eating 75 grams of protein per day. It is not necessary to analyze and/or quantitate protein intake on a regular basis because most people get enough. For reference, 3-4 square meals per day that contain at least one high quality protein food (eggs, chicken, meat, etc.) will meet your daily protein requirement. For those looking to increase protein intake, start by simply taking larger portions of the protein food with each meal (a three- instead of two-egg omelette for breakfast, or an additional half serving of grilled chicken with dinner, etc.)... Another option is to add in a protein supplement (more on this later).

There is one instance where monitoring protein intake takes on great importance: weight loss diets. If you are trying to lose weight, it is critical to be mindful of your protein intake. In general, and as outlined above, most diets are based on eating less *of something*. That is still true, but the one thing you should *not* be eating less of is protein. Protein is used for a variety of purposes in your body, but in a weight loss scenario, it is very important due to its ability to support lean mass. When dieting, the goal is to reduce body fat while maintaining or increasing lean mass (skeletal muscle). Increased dietary protein can accomplish this while also tempering the increased appetite that accompanies many weight loss diets.

Another issue concerning protein intake is dietary displacement. By increasing protein, something else will tend to decrease (this is usually a good thing).   This occurs because protein is very satiating.   Increasing dietary protein for weight loss is a win-win situation, and is supported by clinical research. Not only is dietary protein more satiating, but it also requires more energy to digest and assimilate than carbs.

With regards to the quality of different types of protein, it is fairly simple. Animal proteins, such as milk, cheese, meat, and eggs are complete proteins. They are considered 'high quality.' The proteins found in vegetables are considered 'incomplete' because they are not nutritionally adequate; they lack certain essential amino acids. Vegetarians should consume a variety of different vegetable proteins with each meal in order to provide the body with all of these essential amino acids.

The good: Protein

Increased protein consumption is particularly important during a weight loss diet to avoid losing skeletal muscle. Most diets are intended to reduce fat, not muscle. Muscle is a major component of energy expenditure and supports overall well-being. Muscle wasting, as seen in aging [sarcopenia], cancer [cachexia], very low fat diets, etc., causes many problems: reduced quality of life, increased risk of falling, immobility issues, reduced metabolic rate, etc. Besides supporting muscle mass, dietary protein enhances satiety; it reduces your appetite for an amount of time significantly *longer* than an isocaloric serving of carbohydrates. Some of the longest-term diet studies conducted to date have demonstrated that subjects with the highest protein intake maintained the greatest amount of weight lost.

The exact reason why a high protein intake is associated with weight loss and reduced weight re-gain is unclear, although it has been observed in virtually every population of people in which it has been tested.

Note: weight loss and maintenance of a reduced body weight are two distinct events. Duration of the former is usually less than a year while that of the latter is for the rest of your life. It is much easier to lose weight than to keep it off.

High protein meals require more energy to digest and assimilate, which expends some of the calories eaten (this is another example of how the human body reacts to foods differently than a bomb calorimeter... the bomb calorimeter does not digest and assimilate the meal, it only burns it).

The thermic effect of feeding: total energy expenditure is greater in the hours following a high protein meal relative to an isocaloric high carbohydrate or fat meal. This is not detected by a bomb calorimeter! The difference is too small to be detected in very short studies (as seen below in the study by Weigl), but is likely to become more significant in the long-term.

Protein and appetite

Perhaps it is because high protein foods contain fewer sugars, which, as stated above, makes them less likely to be overeaten. Alternatively, high protein foods may be intrinsically more satiating. This was tested in an interesting study that was designed to examine the effects of increasing protein on appetite, independent of carbohydrates (Weigle, Breen et al. 2005). They tested three diets:

	protein	fat	carbs
baseline	15%	35%	50%
isocaloric	30%	20%	50%
ad lib	30%	20%	50%

This study suffers from its short duration (12 weeks), but the dietary intervention and food intake measurements were very thorough. The nutrient composition of the baseline diet is shown in the table above, and the total calories were adjusted so that each subject was weight stable. This ended up to be, on average, 2300 kilocalories per day. The next phase of the experiment involved feeding an isocaloric, higher protein diet. The subjects maintained their body weight on 2300 kilocalories of the baseline diet, so they were expected to maintain their body weight on the isocaloric higher protein diet. The difference in body weight after the isocaloric diet was less than one pound (statistically non-significant). The isocaloric high protein diet *should have caused* a greater thermic effect of feeding and resulted in increased energy expenditure causing a negative energy balance (and weight loss). Unfortunately, this study lacked the sensitivity to detect what we would have predicted to be a very small difference. In other words, the metabolic boost caused by increasing dietary protein *will* increase energy expenditure, but not enough to result in significant weight loss after only 12 weeks. As discussed above, the 2004 Astrup study demonstrated that high protein diets would indeed promote weight loss but that study was over 1 year long. Lastly, fat mass was not reported so an effect of increased dietary protein on nutrient partitioning cannot be excluded*.

Interestingly, when fed the isocaloric high protein diet, the subjects reported significantly enhanced satiety and reduced hunger. In other words, if they hadn't been instructed to consume *all* of the food they were given, they might have spontaneously eaten less. The researchers tested this by then giving them the same diet but instructed the subjects to eat ad libitum ("at one's pleasure;" or eat as much as desired). Indeed, when given a high protein diet to consume ad libitum, the subjects spontaneously ate significantly less (by almost 400 kilocalories!) and lost weight. The subjects did not dislike the diet; they were simply more satiated and less hungry. Furthermore, leptin[8] levels were unchanged suggesting an independent, intrinsic, satiating effect of increased dietary protein. Collectively, these findings suggest that one of the mechanisms by which increased dietary protein contributes to weight loss is by causing a spontaneous reduction in food intake.

*These findings were later confirmed in a similar study by Larsen (Larsen, Dalskov et al. 2010). In this study, researchers followed a much larger group of subjects for a longer period of time (26 weeks). Larger subject population + longer study duration = more power to detect small differences. By increasing dietary protein from 17% to 23% of calories, the subjects did indeed lose approximately 2 pounds of fat. Interestingly, they also gained 1 pound muscle which clearly demonstrates a nutrient partitioning effect of

---

[8] Leptin: signals "well-fed" to the brain, among other things

increased dietary protein (more on nutrient partitioning in **Chapter 13**).

This study also included a group that increased their protein intake but also switched to more higher glycemic index carbohydrates. As discussed later, this would increase the amount of insulin secreted after every meal. Insulin inhibits fat loss but promotes muscle building. Thus, as expected, consuming higher glycemic index carbohydrates caused elevated insulin levels, almost completely abrogated the fat loss, but modestly increased the amount of muscle gained. From those changes, it was concluded that insulin inhibits fat loss to a greater degree than it promotes muscle building.

Dietary carbohydrates

Dietary carbohydrates are not essential. However, your body *needs* glucose. An essential nutrient is defined as a nutrient that cannot be synthesized by the body in sufficient quantities. The brain requires approximately 130 grams of glucose every day. This does not need to come from the diet because your liver can easily synthesize that amount in a process known as gluconeogenesis. However, this does not mean that certain carbohydrates have no place in a healthy diet... more importantly, there are some very beneficial nutrients found exclusively in carbohydrate-containing foods (that is, foods that contain little protein or fat). For example, blueberries have high amounts of anti-oxidants and beneficial phytochemicals, can potentially improve cognitive functions, but are practically entirely carbohydrates. Most of the calories in blueberries come from sugar, but the nutrients in blueberries are more health-promoting than the sugars are detrimental (the benefits outweigh the costs). Furthermore, no one became obese by overeating blueberries. This stands in contrast to other dietary staples in certain cultures like rice or pasta. Most pasta (noodles, spaghetti, etc.) contains few vitamins or minerals. They are filling, and certain dishes go very well with pasta (or rice); but strictly nutritionally speaking... empty calories.

Dietary carbohydrates can be broken down into three subclasses: fibres, complex carbohydrates, and simple sugars. Carbs are the most abundant food component [in the world].

Dietary fibre is found primarily in vegetables and is extremely important for digestive health. Lack of sufficient dietary fibre is a causative factor in a plethora of digestive disorders, gastrointestinal problems, and even cancer. Eat your leafy greens! And don't forget broccoli, celery, and mixed nuts! In general, soluble or viscous fibres, and insoluble or fermentable fibres, are equally important. Fibre is indigestible so it is technically devoid of calories. Therefore, if you are counting calories or monitoring your carbohydrate intake, be sure to subtract the fibre. To summarize fibre: eat more of it. Many of the same foods that are high in fibre (spinach, broccoli, nuts, etc.) are low calorie and high in vitamins and minerals... the antithesis of 'empty calories.'

Complex carbohydrates are uber-present in television commercials, almost every grocery store aisle, and consequently, in our diet. They comprise breads, rice, wheat, whole grains, pasta, etc., etc. Basically, complex carbohydrates and simple sugars are metabolized similarly by the body, so the term "sugars" has evolved to mean all non-fibre carbohydrates. In other words, nutritionally, carbohydrates can be divided into two, not three, subclasses: fibres and sugars. The important players in the category of simple sugars are glucose (dextrose) and fructose (discussed further below).

Complex carbohydrates are digested into simple sugars within the GI tract. The major difference between complex carbohydrates and simple sugars is that it takes slightly longer for complex carbohydrates to be digested, resulting in a reduced surge in blood glucose compared to simple sugars. Thus, complex carbohydrates have a lower glycemic index value than simple sugars.

The glycemic index, in brief:

- Simple sugars have a higher glycemic index than complex carbohydrates

- Fats, proteins, and fibres, all have a significantly lower glycemic index than complex carbohydrates and simple sugars.

- High blood glucose is bad for you.

- While having no major effect on body weight, low glycemic index diets are usually associated with reduced disease risks and are healthier than high glycemic index diets.

- The easiest low glycemic index diet consists of dietary proteins, fats, and fibres, and is low in all sugars.

- Without any carbohydrates, the glycemic index of a meal is negligible.

Avoid sugars- especially processed foods and added sugars (look for sugars or syrup on food labels). The abundance of high sugar foods in the interior portions of the grocery store is one of the major reasons why it's safer [healthier] to do the bulk of your grocery shopping in the periphery of the grocery store (in other words, don't enter the aisles unless you have to). The best way to reduce sugar consumption is to keep it out of the house! (it ALL starts with the grocery store!)

In sum: Blueberries, leafy greens, and broccoli are examples of healthy carbohydrates. Most juices, snacks, and junk foods, and even staples like rice and pasta have very few vitamins or minerals per calorie and are known as "empty calories."

The bad: Sugars

Dietary sugars are notorious. For optimum health, avoid at all costs. There are, however, some practical reasons to group *all* carbohydrates together when considering energy balance.

1) removal of *all* carbohydrates (not just simple sugars), as seen in certain "low-carb" diets is associated with great weight loss success

2) drugs that block the digestion of complex carbohydrates [modestly] promote weight loss.

The latter point is important and rather complicated. "Alpha-glucosidase" is an enzyme present in the saliva and gastrointestinal tract which breaks down complex carbohydrates. Complex carbohydrates cannot be absorbed intact; they must be degraded first. Drugs that inhibit alpha-glucosidase (e.g., acarbose) block the digestion of complex carbohydrates but have no direct effect on dietary simple sugars ... if simple sugars were the sole culprit, then selectively blocking complex carbs would have no effect. But this is not what happens. Blocking the digestion of complex carbohydrates modestly enhances weight loss.

It should be noted, however, that the effect of alpha-glucosidase inhibitors *alone* on body weight is not robust. These drugs primarily target hyperglycemia, which they treat well. Treatment of an obese insulin resistant population for *three years* led to about a 4 pound weight loss compared to a 1 pound weight gain in the control group (Chiasson, Josse et al. 2003). This study warrants mentioning for its duration; a three-year trial is rare and provides extremely valuable information. In 3 or 6 month studies, there are transient effects; any changes don't really reflect a new set point because a steady state is rarely reached in such a short interval. After three years, however, even if the changes are small, they reflect important, *qualitative* differences that should be viewed with considerably more gravitas than results from a 3 or 6 month-long study.

The findings mentioned above should not be surprising because there was no caloric restriction. In other words, neither carbohydrates nor calories were reduced. Although alpha-glucosidase inhibitors are helpful to mitigate some of the pathological effects of excess dietary carbohydrates, they may be compared to bringing a bucket of water to a forest fire. But this doesn't mean there is nothing to learn here. Actually, *because* alpha-glucosidase inhibitors are not more effective for weight loss, we can make certain inferences into the underlying biology.

Alpha-glucosidase inhibitors do not prevent the digestion of complex carbohydrates, they simply slow it down. In other words, the same amount of carbohydrates will ultimately be absorbed. Carbs are usually digested and absorbed in the small intestine. The major side effect of alpha-glucosidase inhibition is gas and bloating because the carbohydrates now make it all the way to the large intestine. Here they are devoured by the intestinal flora which produces volatile short-chain fatty acids and gas. To be clear: alpha-glucosidase inhibition does not directly reduce energy intake or the total amount of carbohydrates that are absorbed.

Is it possible that alpha-glucosidase inhibitors reduce body weight without altering energy balance?

1) Probably not.

2) if it's true, then the effect is expected to be very small. How small?

4) 4 pounds of fat tissue = ~14,000 kilocalories / 3 years (1095 days) = a mere 13 kilocalories per day. This amount of heat is undetectable by even the most sophisticated equipment.

The effect is simply not big enough to question the rules of energy balance. In other words, it contributes little to the calorie debate. However, we *can* say that hyperglycemia and hyperinsulinemia (both of which are reduced by alpha-glucosidase inhibition) are involved in weight gain. Although physiologically they are tightly related, if considered separately as independent variables, glycemia and insulinemia may contribute less to adiposity than total carbohydrate intake.

This theory is indirectly confirmed by the results from dietary intervention trials examining the effects of high and low glycemic index diets on body weight. To be clear, alpha-glucosidase inhibitors artificially reduce the glycemic index of a diet (I say 'artificial' because the 'natural' way would be to eat less glucose). Neither alpha-glucosidase inhibition nor low glycemic index diets produce nearly as much weight loss as carbohydrate restriction. Even if a low glycemic index diet or alpha-glucosidase inhibitor were to produce a similar degree of blood glucose control, it would not be as beneficial as carbohydrate restriction for weight loss.

Dietary fat

The phrase "you are what you eat" is funny, somewhat cryptic, and at least partly true in a nutritional sense. We are made of water, protein, fat, and minerals. Most bodily tissues are continuously broken down and re-built, or 'remodeled.' The basic building blocks for these biosynthetic processes are derived from metabolites and heat produced after food is digested. The fat, however, is quite a different story altogether. The fat in your hips, butt, and thighs is almost exclusively as it was when you ate it. In other words, analysis of the fats from an adipose tissue biopsy can provide researchers with detailed information about their subject's dietary patterns. The proteins in our body, on the other hand, are not qualitatively affected by the type of proteins in our diet. Thus, with regard to fat, the old adage 'you are what you eat' holds true.

Dietary fat is essential. That means it is necessary to sustain life. Of course, fat is a valuable source of energy as well, but the benefits of consuming high quality fats go far beyond that. First, a definition of what is meant by the 'quality' of fats: dietary fats can be divided into 2 subtypes: saturated and unsaturated. Unsaturated fatty acids are further divided into polyunsaturated omega-3 and omega-6, and monounsaturated omega-9. For the sake of simplicity: vegetable oils are primarily omega-6; in the diet they are usually industrially modified, are pro-inflammatory, and are generally considered to be bad for you. Foods artificially enriched in omega-6 are usually processed foods and should be avoided whenever possible (check food labels, ingredients lists, etc.). Furthermore, omega-6 fats are a major source of the dreaded industrial lipotoxins "trans-fats," which are associated with just about every disease and morbidity experienced by mankind (more on trans fats below).

To reiterate: vegetable oils are primarily omega-6, and the ones found in the diet are usually industrially modified and are unhealthy. The only major exception to the vegetable oil/omega-6 rule is olive oil, which contains a lot of omega-9 fatty acids, and is good for you (or "health neutral"). Avoid vegetable oils, except for olive oil. A beneficial side effect of avoiding vegetable oils is that you will be minimizing your exposure to the dreaded trans-fats and most processed foods (can we call this "collateral reparation?"). Examples of vegetable oils are canola oil, soybean oil, safflower oil, and rapeseed/canola oil. What to use instead?

Go back in time to what they used to use in *the good old days*: butter or lard. A secret weapon guaranteed to get almost anyone to enjoy eating vegetables: sauté them in bacon fat! One or two tablespoons of bacon grease will do wonders to sauté a pound of asparagus stalks or chopped peppers.

One last note, or a disclaimer: natural, native vegetable oil-derived omega-6 fatty acids may not be as bad as the vegetable oil-derived omega-6 fatty acids found in the diet. A lot of the vegetable oils in our diet have been industrially modified, which changes the chemical characteristics of the oil and also the molecular structure of its constituent fatty acids. Actually, we might even be deficient in natural, unmodified omega-6 fatty acids! To be clear, reducing omega-6 fatty acid intake might be healthful because in practice, this is primarily accomplished by avoiding processed foods which simultaneously reduces refined grain *and* trans fat consumption.

Moving on...

Saturated fatty acids, like those found in most animal products, are generally health neutral. They have a longer shelf-life than most fats and therefore do not become rancid. Saturated fatty acids cannot be converted into the dreaded trans-fats, nor can they be 'oxidized.'

Oxidation: remember anti-oxidants? Foods like green tea and blueberries are very high in anti-oxidants. Other examples of anti-oxidants are Vitamins C and E. The role of anti-oxidants in our body is to prevent or reverse malevolent oxidative processes. One such group of molecules that are susceptible to oxidation is unsaturated fatty acids. Upon oxidation, unsaturated fatty acids become rancid and trigger free radical damage, producing harmful effects in the tissues of your body. Important: saturated fatty acids are the least oxidizable of all of the major dietary fatty acids.

Polyunsaturated fatty acids are susceptible to oxidation, can become trans fats, and are pro-inflammatory. There is one exception, however, to the close relationship between unsaturated fatty acids and unhealthiness. That is fish oils. Fish oils are technically very long chain polyunsaturated omega-3 fatty acids, and they provide a host of health benefits. Fish oil supplements are OK, although most of the strongest data in support of the health-promoting aspects of fatty fish consumption came from observing the astounding lack of disease in people who actually ate a lot of fatty fish (like salmon and tuna). The two major fatty acids in fish oil are eicosapentaenoic acid (EPA) and docosahexaenoic acid (DHA). You don't need to know these, just eat fatty fish! If you really can't do it, look for a high quality fish oil supplement such as Barlean's or Carlson's, or ask your doctor about prescription Lovaza. The formal recommendation is to consume fish, but it is better to use a high quality supplement than to miss out on benefits of fish oils. Your entire family will benefit from fish oils- they support and enhance cardiovascular, immune, and mental health (and much more). Fish oils are beneficial for children with attention-deficit hyperactivity disorder, and have even been shown to reduce violent and oppositional behavior. Fish oils elevate mood and improve cognition.

To summarize, saturated fats (like those found in butter & red meat) and fish oils (salmon, tuna, krill, etc.) are good. Vegetable oils are bad, except olive oil. Sugar should be minimized or avoided.

Last but not least, it is safe to say that low-saturated fat and cholesterol-free food products offer no health benefits. This may go against much popular belief, but the negative perception of these two dietary lipids is over-hyped and not supported by the evidence. Cholesterol and saturated fats serve many vital biological functions and are synthesized by every tissue in your body. They are not bad for you (see below).

This has been known for quite some time, but for reasons that have been discussed at great length by authors better than me, the wrong message prevailed ("whoever speaks loudest gets their message heard?"). The relationship between a variety of dietary factors and mortality has been investigated on very large scales, in enormous studies that have cost millions of dollars. In one of the most important diet studies, the Framingham Heart Health Study, investigators tried to figure out if serum cholesterol and heart disease could be related to any of five dietary factors: calories, animal fat, vegetable fat, protein, or cholesterol. They used food frequency questionnaires to acquire food intake data in more than 5,000 residents of Framingham, Massachusetts. In general, the food frequency questionnaire is an inferior technique to determine food intake; however, in this case, the researchers were *extremely* thorough. And anyway, they really only wanted to know about those 5 factors. This study began in the 1950's and is still running.

To make a long story short, almost every finding of the Framingham study was a surprise to the investigators. For example, they found that a higher calorie intake was associated with modestly lower serum cholesterol. You may have thought that people with a higher calorie intake might exercise more, which could potentially explain their lower cholesterol levels. Nope, the inverse relationship between calories and serum cholesterol was true regardless of physical activity levels. Total dietary fat intake usually tracks well with calorie intake, and this held true; higher fat intake was associated with slightly lower cholesterols levels. Protein? No relationship. Dietary cholesterol? No relationship. Basically, in one of the biggest epidemiological studies of all time, they found pretty much no relationship between calories, fat, protein, or dietary cholesterol with serum cholesterol and heart disease. Some have concluded that they simply failed to detect significant relationships. Unlikely. The director of the Framingham study said: *"...the more saturated fat one ate, the more cholesterol one ate, the more calories one ate, the lower the person's serum cholesterol ... the people who ate the most cholesterol, ate the most saturated fat, ate the most calories, weighed the least and were the most physically active[9]"* (Castelli 1992). While those conclusions are sure to provide fuel for conspiracy theories, the most appropriate conclusion should be that the Framingham Study proved serum cholesterol and heart disease are not caused by too much or too little calories, fat, protein, or dietary cholesterol.

"Mr. FIT" (Multiple Risk Factor Intervention Trial) was another great study that came to a similarly surprising result. In this massive intervention study, which included over 12,000 men, a lifestyle intervention consisting of reduced saturated fat and cholesterol intake (among other things) was compared to a 'standard care' control group. To make a long story short, those seemingly healthy lifestyle choices were actually associated with a higher risk of all-cause mortality compared to the standard care.

Many of the biggest and most expensive studies in nutritional sciences consistently report the same thing: the amount of dietary cholesterol or saturated fat does not predict all-cause mortality. Saturated fat and cholesterol are not bad for you. Trans fats, on the other hand, are.

---

[9] William Castelli, 1992

Trans fats

Trans fats are everywhere. Go to your cupboards; grab any packaged foods like crackers or a box of cereal and you will find the words "partially hydrogenated" or "fractionated" in the ingredients list. So, what are trans fats and how bad for you are they?

There are two types of fatty acids: saturated (no double bonds) and unsaturated (1 or more double bonds). Fatty acids can be relatively straight molecules, except double bonds in the "cis" configuration put a "kink" in them. "Cis" is the opposite of "trans;" saturated fats are neither cis nor trans because they don't have any double bonds. Trans fats are **exactly** like unsaturated fats except the kink is straightened out a bit. So trans fats have 1 or more double bond, like unsaturated fats, but are relatively straight, like saturated fats.

It's kind of amazing that these molecules are so similar, yet you can eat 150 grams of saturated and cis-unsaturated fats every day and live a long healthy life, or eat 5 grams of trans fats, become obese and die prematurely.

Trans fats start out as liquid cis-unsaturated fats in vegetable oils (e.g., soybean oil, canola oil, etc.). From a manufacturing standpoint, cis-unsaturated fats are too soft and unstable. So to put them into foods would result in a messy product that melted at room temperature and went rancid in just a few days. That is not exactly what you think of when you picture a delicious warm breakfast muffin, some crispy crackers, or a crème-filled cookie. Converting cis-unsaturated fats into trans-unsaturated fats is what makes the difference. Now your favorite breakfast food has the perfect consistency, tastes delicious, and doesn't go bad. From the perspective of the food company, people will buy more because it tastes better, and they don't have to worry about it going stale if there is a slump in sales. Win-win... except they are very bad for you.

The Nurses' Health Study began in the mid-70's and has been steadily collecting data on over 100,000 women. One seminal manuscript from that study critically examined the effect of dietary trans fats on coronary heart disease (Hu, Stampfer et al. 1997). They analyzed data from roughly 80,000 women, an exorbitant amount of subjects.

On average, 2.2% of the total ingested calories came from trans fat. That's about 5 grams on a 2,000 kcal diet. Average total fat intake was 37.1% of total calories, or 82 grams per day, so trans fats comprised about 6% of the total fat intake.

The first analysis tested for correlations between different fats. Basically, they found that trans fat intake correlated much better with polyunsaturated and monounsaturated fat than with saturated fat. That should be at least partially expected, because trans fats *are* unsaturated fats; so by definition if you're eating more trans fat then you're eating more unsaturated fat. You might have thought that unhealthy people eat a lot of saturated *and* trans fat, so those two things should have correlated better. But they didn't. It appears as though there are some people who eat vegetable oils and trans fats while others eat saturated fats. There is of course much overlap, but that's the gist of the first analysis.

Next they broke it down further. Cholesterol and saturated fats are virtually always found in the same foods (animal products). Therefore, people who ate the least saturated fat also ate the least cholesterol, and people who ate the most saturated fat also ate the most cholesterol. Trans fats come from vegetable oils, and there is no cholesterol in vegetable oils; thus, people who ate the least trans fats also ate the most cholesterol, and people who ate the most trans fat also ate the least cholesterol.

Healthy people try to avoid both saturated and trans fats, and healthy people who eat the least saturated and trans fat were also found to eat the most fibre (probably because they think it contributes to their good health). People who eat the least saturated or trans fats also exercise the most, smoke the least, etc.

When comparing dietary fat intake levels with coronary heart disease, trans fat was the absolute highest risk factor. For the highest quintile of trans fat intake compared to the lowest, relative risk was 1.53; in other words, women who consumed 2.9% of total calories as trans fats (~8 grams per day) had a 53% greater chance of developing coronary heart disease than those who consumed 1.3% of total calories as trans fats (~2.9 grams). A difference of only 5 grams per day increased their risk by half! Where can 5 grams of trans fat hide? 1 serving of French fries, chicken nuggets, 3 slices of pizza, 1 ½ doughnuts, a muffin, a few crackers, ½ bag of microwave popcorn, etc., etc.

Furthermore, the Nurses' Health Study also demonstrated some interesting facts about other dietary fats. The age-adjusted risk for the highest saturated fat intake (18.8% of total calories or ~41 grams per day) compared to the lowest (10.7% or 24 grams) was pretty high: 1.38, or a 38% greater risk of coronary heart disease. However, *some* unhealthy people do indeed eat a lot of saturated fat *and* trans fats. Trans fat is the real bad guy, so when the researchers statistically controlled for trans fat intake, they found that the eating a lot of saturated fat no longer increased risk for coronary heart disease. Not surprisingly, since animal fats are primarily saturated fats, the same thing happened for animal fat consumption. The risk for coronary heart disease in the highest animal fat intake group versus the lowest was 1.30; but after it was adjusted for trans fat the risk went to 0.97 which technically means that a high consumption of animal fat is protective (a 3% lower risk of coronary heart disease). But the result was statistically non-significant, so we conclude: the risk for coronary heart disease is not affected by saturated fat or animal fat intake. Since cholesterol intake does *not* correlate with trans fat intake, there was no association between dietary cholesterol and risk for coronary heart disease before or after adjusting for trans fat intake.

In sum, MrFIT, Framingham, and the Nurses' Health Study all came to similar conclusions: saturated fats and cholesterol are not bad for you.

SATURATED

animal	plant
dairy	coconut oil
eggs	palm oil
red meat	cocoa butter

UNSATURATED

MUFA		PUFA	
animal	plant	animal	plant
poultry	olive oil	fish	corn oil
	avocado		soybean oil
			trans fats

What the heck kind of vegetable produces oil?   When it comes to optimal nutrition, the answer should be "none."

GOOD FATs

saturated   unsaturated

eggs
steak
dairy

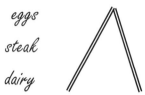

omega-3 & 9   fish oils

olive oil   *salmon*

BAD FATs

unsaturated

omega-6   trans fat

canola   *French fries*

soybean   *hydrogenated*

packaged or processed foods

Saturated *(steak, eggs, dairy)*

Unsaturated

   Monounsaturated: omega-9 *(olive oil)*

   Polyunsaturated

      Omega-3 *(fish oil)*

      Omega-6

         vegetable oils *(canola)*

         trans fats *(hydrogenated)*

The not-so-bad after-all: Fat and satiety

Dietary fat promotes satiety and contains essential fatty acids, which are, well, essential. In fact, both protein *and* fat are essential. Interestingly, fat does not taste very good. How much olive oil or butter can you eat in one sitting? Not much. But mix in some sugar and you have delicious cake icing. Sugars mixed with almost anything enhances the ability of that food to override the normal "meal termination" signals, and thus promote over eating.

After a hearty salad, well-marbled steak, and some grilled asparagus stalks, you would probably feel full. Very full. So full that you couldn't take another bite... However, you could easily have some dessert, a bowl of ice cream or a few cookies perhaps. If you skipped dessert, you would not be hungry later; and having eaten the dessert doesn't make you any more satiated.

The dinner itself was not "over-eaten." When the carb-rich dessert was added, even though the bulk of the calories came from the steak, **the dessert *caused* the positive energy balance** because it is easy to over eat carb-rich foods.

Paradoxes galore

<u>The French Paradox</u>: The French consume significantly more saturated fat than Americans but have much less heart disease. The French Paradox was born in 1987 (Richard 1987).

The French people get more of their fat from animal sources than Americans. They eat approximately 72 grams of animal fat per day compared to about 108 grams for Americans, and slightly more total fat (171 vs. 157). The French eat more cheese and significantly more pork than Americans. In other words, the French eat a lot of saturated fat. Americans consume significantly more polyunsaturated fat than the French, but death from heart disease is approximately 38% greater for Americans.

Some have attributed this to red wine; the French drink more red wine than Americans. While the relationship between red wine and heart disease doesn't hold up in many other nations, this hasn't stopped people from attributing the French paradox to red wine.

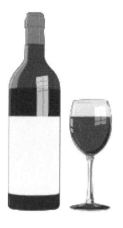

However, the abundance of omega-6 fats in the American diet is the more likely culprit. I'm not saying "don't drink red wine," I'm saying "eat less processed vegetable oils." (this conclusion is in no way influenced by my adoration for red wine.)

An additional pseudo-paradox, known as the Alpine Paradox (Hauswirth, Scheeder et al. 2004), refutes the notion that red wine explains the French paradox. This was not a genuine diet study, but rather a set of observations. The Swiss people consume a high fat diet like the French, but also have low heart disease mortality[10]. However, the Swiss people drink significantly less red wine than the French. Some have attributed this to the specific dairy fats in genuine Swiss cheese. In any case, this is another example of a dissociation between a high saturated fat diet and cardiovascular mortality.

---

[10] World Health Organization, 2000

The American Paradox: Atherosclerosis progresses faster in people who eat less saturated fat than in those who eat more.

In the Mozaffarian study (Mozaffarian, Rimm et al. 2004), researchers capitalized on a technique known as "coronary angiography." As an atherosclerotic plaque develops within the vasculature, the circumference of the blood vessel through that region is decreased. This can be quantified by coronary angiography. The researchers performed this technique on a group of 235 women, then measured food intake and dietary patterns, followed the women for 3.1 years, and finally repeated the coronary angiography.

At first, you might think this study will not provide very accurate results because 235 is too small of a sample size. It is not. The study was very long-term (3.1 years) and the results were acquired using extremely precise instrumentation; these factors drastically increase the statistical power of this study. Moreover, this study was *prospective*, meaning that it followed its subjects over a period of time, as opposed to collecting all the data retrospectively. Retrospective studies are subject to significantly more confounding than prospective studies.

Back to the data: total saturated fat intake ranged from 5% to 13% of total calories (14 – 36 grams per day on a 2,500 kilocalorie diet). The women who ate the most saturated fat also ate the most cholesterol (because they are found in the same foods). The arteries in women who ate the least saturated fat got a little bit narrower over the course of the study. This is not really unexpected because atherosclerosis is a progressive disease, and it was simply progressing in these subjects. The surprise came when the researchers found that arteries in women who ate the most saturated fat didn't get any smaller at all. And there was a linear effect: the less saturated fat in the diet, the more atherosclerosis would progress in the arteries. The American paradox was born in 2004.

The American paradox shouldn't really be thought of as a paradox. Saturated fat is one of the few things known to increase the good cholesterol (high density lipoprotein, HDL). High HDL is theorized to function, at least in part, by to trafficking cholesterol *out* of the body. Thus, high HDL levels, achieved by consuming a diet rich in saturated fat, should have been predicted to reduce the progression of atherosclerosis. This could very well explain the American paradox.

However, another interesting finding emerged from this study. The exact opposite trend was seen for carbohydrates. In other words, a high intake of dietary carbohydrates was directly associated with greater progression of atherosclerosis. You may have heard some dietary advice along the lines of "reduce your fat intake, specifically saturated fats; and eat more healthy carbohydrates for a heart healthy diet." The results from the Mozaffarian study state, categorically, this advice is wrong.

The standard disclaimer: this study was not a randomized intervention trial. It was observational and therefore cannot definitely establish a cause and effect relationship. The HDL connection provides biological plausibility, but does serve as evidence of causation. Determining a true cause and effect would require taking a group of subjects and giving half of them a treatment that you think will cause atherosclerosis (a low saturated fat high carbohydrate diet), which is unethical. A statistical analysis of the results showed that the enhanced atherosclerotic progression was *most likely* due to the reduced saturated fat intake because the relationship was true in a wide variety of subjects, regardless of their physical activity, tobacco use, body weight, etc.

A paradox? I think not.

The Spanish Paradox: Increasing consumption of red meat and fish while decreasing consumption of wheat, whole grains, and carbohydrate-rich foods resulted in reduced mortality from heart disease and stroke.

In 1966, a group of researchers in Spain began gathering basic food intake data (Serra-Majem, Ribas et al. 1995). They asked a large cohort of Spaniards about their usual intake of meat, dairy, fish, oils, grains, sugars, etc. In 1990, 24 years later, they did it again. In the meantime, they recorded health outcomes and causes of death for each study participant. Between 1966 and 1990 they found a linear increase in the amount of meat, dairy, fish and berries consumed, and a decrease in vegetable oils, whole grains, and many carbohydrate-rich foods. They also observed a large reduction in heart disease and stroke mortality.

No sirs, these are not paradoxes.

<u>another notable paradox (it's more of an
'exception' than a bona fide paradox)</u>

There may be multiple factors that
contribute to the development of obesity. Some
factors might be more or less important in different
contexts. The majority of this book has put the
most blame on processed foods, grains, and a high
carbohydrate diet. That is because in Western
society, these are the most important factors. This
is not always the case, however.

The average Western diet derives
approximately half of its calories from
carbohydrates. The average Westerner is
overweight or obese. Does the Western diet cause
obesity? Which components of the Western diet
are important? These questions are important and
complicated. One way to break down diets is by
macronutrients. For example, the average
Western diet is 55% carbohydrates, 30% fat, and
15% protein. Given the marked success of
carbohydrate restriction in treating obesity, this
population is clearly intolerant to their 55%
carbohydrates. However, the Kitavan people from
Papua, New Guinea consume roughly 70%
carbohydrates and are lean and fit (Lindeberg,
Eliasson et al. 1999). This may be due to a number

of factors. For example, the Kitavan diet is very low in sugar and whole grains. Sugars are easily over-eaten and grains interfere with leptin signaling (Jonsson, Olsson et al. 2005); collectively, these differences could explain why the Kitavans are able to stay lean on 70% carbohydrates. They likely experience postprandial hyperinsulinemia, but this does not result in fat accumulation because the lack of sugars and grains makes them less likely to be insulin resistant and overeat. Actually, they have reduced fasting insulin levels (Lindeberg, Nilsson-Ehle et al. 1994) because of their very high insulin sensitivity.

In this population, it may not be the *quantity* of carbohydrates, but is rather the *quality* that is important. Could Westerners lose weight on 70% carbohydrates if they cut out the sugars and grains? If the diet was significantly hypocaloric, then it's possible. But a diet consisting 70% carbohydrates excluding sugars and grains would be completely foreign to a Westerner. Most would have no idea what to eat!

Furthermore, there are other qualitative differences in the Kitavan diet such as the virtual absence of industrially modified omega-6 polyunsaturated fatty acids. As stated above, omega-6 polyunsaturated fatty acids are pro-inflammatory and reduce insulin sensitivity. The low omega-6 in the Kitavan diet means they are more insulin sensitive and thus more tolerant to a carb-rich diet. OK, so could Westerners lose weight on 70% carbohydrates if they cut out sugars, grains, *and* omega-6 fats? Possibly, but this diet is becoming more and more unfamiliar and is therefore unlikely to be sustainable long-term.

One very important conclusion that can be drawn from comparing the Kitavan and Western diets, however, is that carbohydrates by themselves are not the cause of obesity. If not carbohydrates, then what is causing obesity in Westerners but not Kitavans?

Although Kitavans consume more carbohydrates, Kitavans most likely have lower 24 hour insulin levels than Westerners. Both diets are expected to stimulate insulin *secretion* to a similar degree: the Kitavan due to the sheer quantity of carbohydrates; the Western diet has fewer carbohydrates but a higher glycemic index value. But the Kitavan may not become as hyperglycemic as a Westerner, and their insulin levels will return to baseline sooner because of the low consumption of omega-6 fats and higher insulin sensitivity. So is the higher glycemia that causes obesity in

Westerners? Does this implicate *insulin resistance* rather than total carbohydrates?

Furthermore, the Kitavans may be less likely to overeat because of the low consumption of sugars and grains and higher leptin sensitivity. So does it all come back to energy balance?

These questions are complicated and the answers are far from clear. They cannot be extrapolated from the data, and trying to do so may be very misleading. It is an extreme oversimplification to directly compare these two cultures, and many of the connections that we try to make are primarily speculative. In order to absolutely prove that these correlations are indeed causations would require strictly controlled randomized intervention trials, which will probably never occur. So we are left with logical inferences and educated guesses.

Chapter 8.
Fructose, leptin, et al.

Fructose

Fructose is a simple sugar, similar to glucose except it is comprised of a 5-membered ring instead of 6.

Fructose   Glucose

Fructose is naturally found predominantly in fruits. Fructose is fruit sugar. It is what makes fruit sweet and delicious. This is a very beneficial characteristic for fruits as it promotes seed dispersion. Prior to maturity, fruits are usually bitter and animals stay away. When the seeds mature, however, the fruit ripens and its sugar content increases. Animals eat the sweet fruits; the seeds pass through the digestive tract and are dispersed where ever the animal goes to the bathroom[11]. Historically, humans were also drawn to sweet fruits; we probably like sweet things

---

[11] #2

because ripe fruits are rich in vitamins and minerals. In modern times, however, most of the fructose in the diet comes from table sugar. The average person consumes over 60 pounds of fructose a year, predominantly from table sugar and high fructose corn syrup (discussed below). Table sugar is predominantly sucrose, a "disaccharide" comprised of glucose and fructose.

Sucrose

The most malevolent form of fructose is found in corn syrup, or more specifically, high-fructose corn syrup. This is the sweetener found in most processed foods, in everything from bread to soft drinks to breakfast cereals. It is cheap and very sweet.

Unlike glucose, fructose does not trigger an insulin response. Does this mean it's healthier than glucose? No, not even close. Unlike glucose, which can be utilized by almost every cell of the body, the only tissue that can sufficiently metabolize fructose is the liver. When excess glucose floods into the liver, flux through the metabolic pathways is moderated by key regulatory enzymes. Fructose, on the other hand, bypasses many of these enzymes. One consequence of this is phosphate depletion, which is a direct insult to the liver. This is why fructose administered intravenously will cause liver failure in a matter of minutes. In other words, fructose can be toxic.

Another consequence of this is that excess fructose carbons flood into lipogenic pathways. That means instead of being oxidized, stored, or exported, fructose gets incorporated into lipids. Being that this takes place in the liver, and given that fructose is easily over-eaten, the resulting positive energy balance is invested in <u>hepatic</u> fat deposition. In other words, it is a ticket to non-alcoholic fatty liver disease (NAFLD). A fatty liver is a dysfunctional and insulin resistant liver. As such, NAFLD is one of the earliest steps in the etiology of the metabolic syndrome. It is quite possible that fructose-induced NAFLD and the subsequent hepatic insulin resistance are the major culprits in precipitating the downward spiral to frank carbohydrate intolerance and insulin resistance, and ultimately to obesity and type II diabetes.

There are interesting theories on the relative contribution of fructose to the obesity epidemic. Some believe that limiting fructose consumption to that found in whole foods (fruits) would have drastic effects on body weight control. This scenario posits that fructose-induced NAFLD and subsequent hepatic insulin resistance cause hyperglycemia, which causes insulin resistance and hyperinsulinemia. The hyperinsulinemia then stimulates the expansion of fat tissue and leptin resistance. In other words, without the initial insult (fructose), dietary carbohydrates would never cause a problem because the body would be insulin sensitive. This theory is comprehensive, but fails because of the existence of populations of obese insulin resistant people who consume little fructose. Furthermore, by failing to mention energy balance, the theory implies that obesity can occur in a hypocaloric state. Fructose may increase your susceptibility to diet-induced obesity, but is neither necessary nor sufficient to *cause* obesity. In other words, fructose *can* have a major role, but it is not acting alone.

Leptin

Leptin is secreted from fat cells and sends a "well-fed" signal to the brain. Leptin levels are correlated with absolute levels of body fat and *changes in body fat*. The more adipose tissue you have, the higher your leptin levels will be. Moreover, leptin levels are also elevated by overfeeding (when body fat is expected to increase). The opposite is also true: lean people have lower leptin levels than obese; and fasting or calorie restriction markedly lowers leptin levels.

OK, so leptin basically tracks with body fat, what does it do? Leptin tells the brain that the body is well-fed and has plenty of energy stored up, it is OK to stop foraging for food and start playing. Obese people have excess fat mass and, accordingly, very high leptin levels. So why isn't leptin signaling "well-fed" to their brain? It is postulated that obese insulin-resistant patients are leptin-resistant and therefore may be more hungry and tired. At present, there appears to be a very close relationship between insulin resistance and leptin resistance.

For a while, researchers were baffled as to why leptin injections didn't reduce appetite in obese subjects. Eventually, this was passively chalked up to leptin resistance. But later on, however, it was discovered that low leptin may actually be a more important signal of starvation than high leptin is a signal of being well-fed. In other words, lowering leptin levels, as seen during starvation, is a more potent signal than increasing leptin, as seen during overfeeding or weight gain. In other words, leptin will make you hungry and prepare you for starvation in times of energy deficit to a greater degree than it will tell you to stop eating in times of energy excess. Much of this was teased out in one very clever study[12].

When the body is experiencing an energy deficit, metabolic rate is reduced in order to attenuate the negative energy balance. In a seminal paper by Rosenbaum and colleagues (Rosenbaum, Goldsmith et al. 2005), the role of leptin in energy balance was empirically investigated. They performed a battery of metabolic, autonomic, and neuroendocrine tests to 10 patients when they were 1) weight-stable, 2) after losing 10 % of their body weight, and 3) after losing 10 % and then receiving leptin injections. Recall that weight loss reduces leptin levels; thus the researchers administered enough leptin in the 3rd group to achieve plasma leptin levels equivalent

---

[12] IMHO one of the most important papers about leptin

to pre-weight loss levels. As expected, both fat mass and fat-free mass were reduced after weight loss, as was total energy expenditure. The reduction in energy expenditure, as discussed in previous chapters, is *partially* due to the reduction in fat-free mass. The reduction in energy expenditure is also *partially* caused by an increase in skeletal muscle efficiency. In other words, muscle is capable of extracting *more* energy from a gram of fat or carbohydrate during starvation (it wastes less energy). This is another example of the discordance between calorimetry and biology. Muscle burns fuel more efficiently when it is in 'starvation mode.' A bomb calorimeter does not have 'starvation mode!'

The interesting part of the study was what happened when leptin was administered to the weight-reduced patients. Leptin administration increased metabolic rate and restored skeletal muscle efficiency to pre-weight loss levels. These results suggest that leptin is the cause for the slowing of weight loss during prolonged diets. In other words, if your baseline energy expenditure was 2,000 kilocalories per day, and you were losing 1 pound a week by consuming 1,500 kilocalories per day, soon you will be losing less than one pound per week in part because leptin has plummeted!

It is also interesting to note *which* component of energy expenditure was affected by weight loss. In general, a reduction in fat-free mass is expected to decrease energy expenditure. These researchers demonstrated that non-resting energy expenditure was reduced *beyond that predicted* by changes in fat-free mass. In other words, skeletal muscle efficiency only matters when skeletal muscle is active. This component was completely restored by leptin. So, theoretically, it could be extrapolated that the effects of reduced leptin levels on energy expenditure can be attenuated by staying in bed…

In contrast to leptin dynamics in a state of energy deficit, insulin stimulates the secretion of leptin during times of energy excess. Since fructose doesn't stimulate insulin secretion, it has been hypothesized that the calories from fructose are not properly relayed to the brain's satiety system (via leptin). Furthermore, it is logical to assume that leptin acts to stimulate energy expenditure, even to the degree of reducing skeletal muscle efficiency in order to burn off additional calories during times of energy surplus. Unless those additional calories are from fructose, because fructose causes a lower secretion of leptin compared to an isocaloric amount of glucose. Thus, fructose may promote over-eating to a greater degree than glucose.

Ghrelin, a stomach-derived hormone thought to be involved in meal initiation, is increased before mealtimes and decreased immediately after. Interestingly, ghrelin levels don't decline as much if the meal contained a lot of fructose. Taken together, these theories suggest that fructose may contribute to passive overconsumption and a positive energy balance by failing to sufficiently induce leptin and suppress ghrelin. Although much is still only theoretical, epidemiological studies have demonstrated a near linear relationship between fructose ingestion and body weight, especially in children.

A note on "perspective."

A high fructose meal may be less
satiating, but not by much. You won't
gain 5 pounds a week by drinking juice
instead of water with breakfast. The
effects of fructose on satiety are expected
to be small (10 kilocalories a day?).
Scientifically, this is a problem. It means
that in order to detect an effect, an
extremely large sample size studied over
an extended period of time is necessary.
This is cost-limiting. We know obesity
doesn't happen overnight, but this is the
only type of study that would provide
unequivocal results.

Here's a curious paradox: if you give a 5-year-old child a cookie, what happens? He bounces off the walls. Referred to in the vernacular as the "sugar high," this is actually the negative feedback system of energy balance at work. But if you give an obese 5-year-old child a cookie, what happens? The child is in the pantry looking for more cookies... The reason for this paradox can be described in 2 words: "leptin resistance[13]" (Lustig 2008). There is probably little truth to that anecdote, but just to

---

[13] Lustig, Robert (2008)

further the point about "perspective," the difference between those two children would not be nearly that dramatic. There *might* be a 10 kilocalorie difference in their behavioral responses to the cookie. It's not what you pictured (a skinny kid running around eating a cookie or a fat kid sitting on the ground with a bowl of cookies). In the quest to find the causative agent responsible for excessive fat accumulation, there will not be a masked villain caught red-handed. We are talking about very small changes. Obesity doesn't happen overnight.

All of these theories about how we over eat have one thing in common that needs to be stressed: they evolve very slowly over time. Given the aforementioned difficulties in assessing energy balance in the laboratory, and the fact that human studies are expensive and relatively short-term, adequately testing these hypotheses is rare. However, the observational, epidemiological, historical, and anecdotal data all agree on one thing: "eat less and move more" is *not* the answer.

It is very possible that estimates of 10 or 20 surplus kilocalories per day to cause obesity in the long-term may actually be accurate. Most human beings are overweight. It is possible that sugars, fructose, and carb-rich meals can indeed promote overconsumption, even if it is only by 10 kilocalories a day. It may seem excessive to abandon the processed food, high-carb lifestyle if it is only going to prevent the overconsumption of 10 kilocalories a day. You be the judge.

10 extra kilocalories a day... it's not as dangerous as playing in traffic

Calories or insulin?

At this point, it is important to be aware of the magnitude of the effects of insulin compared to a positive energy balance. Generally, insulin promotes fat storage, but does this mean you can't lose weight with high insulin levels? No, if the diet is sufficiently hypocaloric then insulin levels will not matter.

For example, an early study by Grey and Kipnis asked a similar question (Grey and Kipnis 1971). In their first experiment, 7 obese subjects were fed for 3 weeks each a low carb diet (25% carbs, 53% fat) then an isocaloric low fat diet (62% carbs, 18% fat). They were weight stable for this portion of the study, and the researchers found that basal insulin levels were decreased by half on the low carb diet and increased by half on the low fat diet. They concluded that high insulin levels are a consequence of specific dietary components, not peripheral insulin resistance (because *all* the subjects were insulin resistant), and then began the second and more important part of the study. In the second experiment, 3 obese subjects engaged in three successive 4-week long hypocaloric 1,500 kcal/d diets; 1st a low fat high carb diet, then a low carb diet, and finally the same low fat high carb diet again. Insulin levels were high in the first period, low in the second, and high again in the final period. Basically, insulin levels tracked with the amount of dietary carbohydrates consumed during each dietary phase. And yes, the subjects lost body weight in all three phases. These results suggest that a sufficient calorie deficit will induce weight loss despite high insulin levels. The study was small (>10 subjects), very short (a few weeks), and did not assess body composition or fat mass, only total body weight. In other words, this study asked a good question, just not the one with which *we* are most interested; the study was not designed to be able to detect if *high insulin levels reduce the rate of fat loss on a hypocaloric diet or if high insulin levels exacerbate fat gain on a hypercaloric diet*. Furthermore, the extent to which the rate of fat loss is reduced by high insulin levels on a hypocaloric diet is expected to be small but significant. In sum, a large degree of calorie restriction is a more powerful determinant of fat loss than low insulin levels; however, with small or no calorie deficits, the role of high insulin in building fat mass will take on a more important role.

While their experiments were pioneering, their interpretation that high insulin levels are a consequence of the diet as opposed to insulin resistance may not have been entirely complete. For example, in a study by Woodhouse and colleagues, 25 overweight sedentary men engaged in an exercise regimen while body weight, diet, and insulin levels were measured (Woodhouse, Sutherland et al. 1984). After one month, body weight and diet were not different from baseline[14]. However, insulin levels immediately plummeted, body fat declined by 16%, and muscle mass increased by 5%! The authors concluded that the changes in body composition were caused by the decline in insulin levels.

The reason why this study is important [right now] is that insulin levels declined despite no change in diet. This stands in contrast to Grey and Kipnis' conclusion that diet, not insulin sensitivity, determines insulin levels. Exercise improves insulin sensitivity, which is the most likely reason why insulin levels dropped in the Woodhouse study. Lower insulin levels promote fat loss, which was also observed in that study. Diet and total calorie

---

[14] The increased energy expenditure from the exercise routine was most likely balanced by a decrease in energy expenditure during the rest of the day. This would maintain energy balance and explain why body weight did not change. But this also suggests that the changes in insulin, not energy balance, were what drove the fat loss.

intake was unchanged, and the added exercise energy expenditure was most likely compensated for by a reduction in non-exercise energy expenditure (the dietary intervention prohibited them from eating more to compensate). **Therefore, they gained muscle, lost fat, and had lower insulin levels despite maintaining energy balance.**

Collectively, the results of these two studies suggest: 1) insulin is regulated both by diet and by insulin sensitivity (Grey and Kipnis; Woodhouse); 2) low insulin levels facilitate fat loss, exercise promotes muscle gain (Woodhouse); 3) it is possible to lose weight with high insulin levels if calories are sufficiently restricted, although the weight lost will be both fat *and* muscle (Grey and Kipnis). Furthermore, these findings present some interesting advantages to weight loss with low insulin levels. Namely, 1) if low insulin levels are achieved via exercise, then muscle mass can be maintained; 2) if low insulin levels are achieved via carbohydrate restriction, then total calories can be unrestricted; and 3) if total calories are unrestricted, then there is a much better chance for an improvement in lean body mass.

Chapter 9.
Rubor, tumor, calor, dolor, functio lasea

"The doctor of the future will no longer treat the human frame with drugs, but rather will cure and prevent disease with nutrition."

Thomas Edison (1847 – 1931)

The title of this chapter is not a spell you'd learn at Hogwarts; they are the cardinal symptoms of inflammation: redness, swelling, heat, pain, and loss of function. Cardiovascular disease, arthritis, hepatitis, bursitis, IBS, and colitis are just a few examples of the inflammatory diseases that plague an alarming amount of people. It is not a stretch to say that inflammation is at the root of most modern diseases. And there is a strong, direct relationship between diet and the induction, maintenance, and resolution of inflammation. Whether or not you are experiencing overt symptoms of inflammation, it would be prudent to consider transitioning to a more anti-inflammatory diet.

Omega-3 and omega-6 fats

With regards to dietary fat, there are two major classes of unsaturated fatty acids that are relevant to inflammation: omega-6 and omega-3. Omega-6 containing fats, in general, are pro-inflammatory, industrially processed, and are the major source of trans fats. These are found in most vegetable oils. Safflower oil, soybean oil, corn oil, and canola oil are all potent sources of omega-6 fats. Read the label of almost any packaged food-like products (breakfast cereals, potato chips, snacks, microwave dinners, etc.) and you will find omega-6 fats.

Omega-3 fatty acids are anti-inflammatory. Salmon, eggs, sardines, tuna, krill and grass-fed beef all contain omega-3 fatty acids. Omega-3 fatty acids compete with omega-6's, which reduces the conversion of omega-6's into pro-inflammatory mediators. AND, in the process, omega-3's become converted into a distinctly different set of anti-inflammatory, or *less pro-inflammatory,* mediators. In sum, the quantity of dietary omega-3 and omega-6 fatty acids impacts the severity of inflammation. Reducing omega-6 and increasing omega-3 can help to ameliorate *excessive* inflammation.

When the body encounters an inflammatory insult, omega-6 fatty acids are converted into pro-inflammatory molecules that usher in the subsequent inflammatory state. This can range from a shoulder pains that only last a week to insulin resistance and diabetes which can last a lifetime. The crucial point is that omega-6 fatty acids come from the diet. The symptoms of inflammatory diseases manifest in a wide range of severity. This variance is due to, in part, the abundance of omega-3 and omega-6 fatty acids available in the body.

Although the health effects of switching to grass-fed beef is yet to be tested, a beneficial effect might be predicted based on the fatty acid composition of grass-fed versus conventional beef. The total omega-3 content of grass-fed beef is significantly greater than grain-fed (7% vs. 1% of the total fatty acids). The ratio of omega-6 to omega-3 in grain-fed beef is 20! The ideal value for this ratio in a healthy diet is 2 to 4 (Simopoulos 2001). For grass-fed beef the value is 1. It's better to go under than over because most commonly eaten foods have a ratio greater than 4; eating grass-fed beef can help to balance it out. If the option is available, request grass-fed-only beef because one trick the farmers use to really fatten up the cattle prior to slaughter is to feed them a ton of grains. At this time in their lives the cattle are accumulating fat mass at an incredible rate, so a lot of the omega-3 fatty acids that accumulated while they were grass-feeding will be diluted by the new grain-based fats. Much of the feed used by farmers is genetically-modified soy. This soy provides a ratio of omega-6 to omega-3 of approximately 60.

> "Let food by thy medicine"
>
> -Hippocrates (ca. 460 BC – ca. 370 BC)

Fish oils

      The most important fatty acids, in terms of inflammatory tone, are arachidonic acid (ARA), eicosapentaenoic acid (EPA), and docosahexaenoic acid (DHA). ARA is a very long chain polyunsaturated omega-6 fatty acid. EPA and DHA are very long chain polyunsaturated omega-3 fatty acids. They are very important. The figure below depicts the major dietary omega-6 and omega-3 fatty acids, linoleic and alpha-linolenic acids, respectively. These are "essential," meaning that they must be acquired via the diet because our body cannot synthesize them [in sufficient quantities]. Although we can synthesize EPA and DHA from alpha-linolenic acid, I deem them to be essential. Essential for what? *That* is the question. If essential means necessary for survival, then maybe DHA and EPA are not as essential as oxygen, but are essential in terms of morbidity and long term mortality risk. I prefer to interpret *essential* more holistically, in that there are great benefits to getting more EPA and DHA than the body can synthesize. And yes, EPA and DHA are my favorite fatty acids.

Omega-6　　　# Omega-3

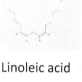

Linoleic acid

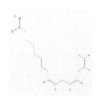

α-Linolenic acid

γ-Linolenic acid
(GLA)

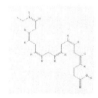

Eicosapentaenoic acid
(EPA)

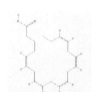

Arachidonic acid
(ARA)

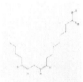

Docosahexaenoic acid
(DHA)

One of the most important clinical endpoints in any clinical trial is mortality. Mortality is known as a "hard endpoint" because there is absolutely no subjectivity to the diagnosis. Subjectivity is involved in declaring the *cause of death*, but not the presence or absence of death. The impact of obesity on longevity has been considerably underestimated because the cause of death is rarely attributed to obesity (an example of subjectivity). A coroner or doctor is much more likely to say sudden cardiac death or myocardial infarction when the true cause was obesity.

Studer and colleagues recently published an article comparing the effects of a variety of different anti-hyperlipidemic agents on mortality (Studer, Briel et al. 2005). Anti-hyperlipidemic drugs are used primarily to treat high blood triacylglycerols (a molecule that is comprised of 3 fatty acids connected to a glycerol backbone) or high cholesterol. To perform this study, or "meta-analysis," the researchers found every study that directly compared a lipid-lowering drug or dietary intervention to placebo and included more than 1,000 subjects.

The treatments were:

1) statins, which decrease cholesterol by around 20%;

2) fibrates, which increase good cholesterol (HDL), decrease bad cholesterol (LDL) by ~8%, and decrease triacylglycerols;

3) omega-3 fatty acids;

4) and dietary interventions.

Right off the bat some strengths of this study are that it excluded any trials that didn't include a placebo group, and included only large-scale trials with over 1,000 subjects. The weakness of this study is not a weakness in how the researchers conducted the study, per se, but rather in the nature of the study. If the outcome of a meta-analysis is controversial, critics will immediately claim that the researchers cherry picked[15] the studies. We can never really know if this is true (if they were intentionally deceitful), but this particular meta-analysis was particularly thorough in its vetting process and still included a lot of big trials.

Of all the treatments, only statins and omega-3 fatty acids significantly reduced all-cause mortality. Out of 35 statin trials which followed patients for an average of 3 years, the overall reduction in mortality was ~13%. This was primarily due to the secondary prevention of coronary heart disease. Secondary prevention means that the patients were prescribed the drug *after* experiencing a major event such as a heart attack. In other words, if you haven't had a heart attack, statins won't do much good. If you have had a heart attack, then statins will decrease your mortality risk by ~13%.

Out of 14 omega-3 trials, which followed patients for an average of 2 years, the overall reduction in mortality was almost twice as good as statins, 25%. This is significant for at least 2 reasons: 1) that is a huge difference, and 2) the studies only lasted 2 years on average, meaning

---

[15] Cherry pick- the derogatory term for including only studies that support your conclusion and selectively excluding any studies that refute your conclusion.

that the benefits of omega-3 fatty acids are fast-onset *and* robust. In other words, statins take ~ 50% longer and are only ~50% as good as omega-3 fatty acids.

Diet was found to be ineffective in this meta-analysis, although I would argue that the actual dietary interventions used in the individual studies were not optimal. Most dietary interventions in the clinical setting are based on large increases in carbohydrate consumption at the expense of fats which, as discussed earlier, is not optimal (especially considering that the most effective reduction in mortality risk came from fats!)

The GSSI-Prevenzione trial was a prospective, secondary prevention trial that compared the effects on mortality of omega-3 fatty acids, vitamin E, both, or neither (Marchioli 1999). The latter two groups are very important. If there was an additional benefit in those who received both, that would indicate a synergistic interaction. In other words, it would mean that both compounds have a distinct mechanism of action. If there no additional benefit to using both, it tends to indicate that the compounds do the same thing. In this case, there was little rationale to suggest that omega-3 fatty acids had a mechanism of action similar to vitamin E. It is likely that the researchers hypothesized a synergistic interaction; vitamin E is a fat-soluble antioxidant and may improve the stability of omega-3 fatty acids, which are theoretically more susceptible to oxidation due to them being *unsaturated* fatty acids.

They recruited over 10,000 patients into the trial, most of them within a month after their first heart attack. The intervention consisted of 880 mg EPA and DHA in a 1:2 ratio, 300 mg vitamin E, or both. That amount of DHA and EPA can be found in about 3 ounces of salmon. 300 mg vitamin E is about 20 times the recommended dose (15 mg) but less than the toxic dose (>1000 mg per day); it is not an uncommon dose in vitamin supplements. After three and a half years, they found that those receiving DHA and EPA had a 15% reduced all-cause mortality compared to placebo. There was no significant effect of vitamin E on mortality, and adding vitamin E to EPA and DHA offered no additional benefit. The findings are in accord with the results of the meta-analysis and further confirm that DHA and EPA may make the difference between life and death.

Statins are the number one prescribed drug of all time and gross an enormous amount of profits for pharmaceutical companies. And practically no one cares for the fish-derived omega-3 fatty acids, EPA and DHA, even though they are a fraction of the cost. Moreover, the very long chain omega-3 fatty acids DHA and EPA do more than prolong lifespan. They promote a better *healthspan*. That is, they improve quality of life. DHA and EPA have been shown to favorably impact mood, cognition, attention, and reduce inflammation in a variety of contexts. In other words, I don't mean to sound 'preachy,' but whether you've had a heart attack or not, it might be a good idea to consider EPA and DHA supplements if you don't like fish. The best sources are whole foods like salmon and tuna, and eggs to a lesser degree, but there are some high quality fish oil supplements available as well. When comparing fish oil supplements, only the EPA and DHA content should be considered, not the total omega-3 content because the benefits of omega-3 fatty acids are due specifically to EPA and DHA.

Nutritionally, EPA and DHA are technically categorized as animal sources of omega-3 fatty acids while α-linolenic acid is a plant source. That is because most EPA and DHA come from fish (even though the fish get it from algae). In general, plants are not an optimal source for dietary fat. Most vegetable oils consist of predominantly pro-inflammatory omega-6 fatty acids and need to have their oils industrially (chemically) extracted. Although alpha-linolenic is a plant-source of omega-3 fats, it is inferior to DHA and EPA.

For example, there is an inducible condition in rats that closely reflects heart failure in humans. Scientists use this model to examine the mechanism of cardiovascular dysfunction in pathological states. In one study, researchers induced heart failure in a group of rats and supplemented them with placebo, α-linolenic acid, or EPA and DHA at three escalating doses (Duda, O'Shea et al. 2009). As expected, supplementation increased the relative content of each fatty acid in the body; that is, α-linolenic acid supplementation increased the α-linolenic acid present in the heart. α-linolenic acid is a precursor to EPA, and supplementation modestly increased the amount of EPA in heart tissue suggesting that either the body converted some of the α-linolenic acid into EPA or supplemental α-linolenic acid has an EPA-sparing effect. EPA is also a precursor to DHA; but α-linolenic acid supplementation did not increase the amount of DHA in heart tissue. This is also seen in humans; the only way to dramatically increase the amount of DHA in the body is by consuming DHA.

To make a long story short, virtually every measurement for heart function was dramatically improved by DHA and EPA, while α-linolenic acid showed little or no effect at all. Many of these findings were found to be due to the pan-anti-inflammatory effects of DHA and EPA.

One of the most famous studies on diet in heart attack patients was the Diet and Reinfarction Trial, or DART (Burr, Fehily et al. 1989). In this secondary prevention trial, over two thousand men who just had their first heart attack were randomly assigned to make one of three changes in their diet and then followed for two years. The interventions were:

1) reduce saturated fat

2) increase fatty fish intake

3) increase cereal fibre

Not surprisingly, reducing saturated fat intake had no effect on mortality. Neither did increasing cereal fibre (which actually increased mortality risk). Consuming just 3 portions of fatty fish (salmon, mackerel, herring, etc.) per week reduced all-cause mortality by 29%.

Saturated fat is one of the only factors known to increase the good cholesterol HDL. High HDL strongly protects against heart disease. The subjects who reduced their saturated fat intake experienced very small reductions in their HDL levels, which may at least partially explain why reducing saturated fat consumption didn't reduce mortality. Moreover, in one study this advice was actually associated with an increase in mortality (Woodhill, Palmer et al. 1978).

Studer's meta-analysis showed us that omega-3 fatty acids were superior to statins in the prevention of all-cause mortality. The GSSI-Prevencione study showed us that the omega-3 fatty acids DHA and EPA were superior to vitamin E and placebo in the prevention of all-cause mortality. Duda's rat study showed us that plant sources of omega-3 fatty acids (α-linolenic acid) were inferior to DHA and EPA. DART showed us that fatty fish consumption markedly reduced all-cause mortality. Collectively, these studies suggest 1) EPA and DHA are the clinically important omega-3 fatty acids, and 2) they are more protective against all-cause mortality than any other known drug on the planet.

The dose of EPA and DHA in GSSI-Prevencione was 880 mg per day, or 6,160 mg per week, and all-cause mortality was reduced by 15%. The dose of EPA and DHA in DART was three servings of fatty fish per week, which would be expected to provide only around 3,000 mg, but the reduction in all-cause mortality, was 29%. Half the dose and twice the benefits. Therefore, while supplementing EPA and DHA in a pill is OK, consuming EPA and DHA in whole foods may be up to 4 times better, milligram for milligram. Exactly why this happens is unclear, but may be due to other protective factors in fatty fish, or possibly just that the whole food source provides for more efficient digestion and absorption of the EPA and DHA. In any case, eat more salmon; it could save your life.

Chapter 10.
Well-fed and stressed out

> Tranquil mind,
> sit like a tortoise,
> walk sprightly like a pigeon,
> sleep like a dog.
>
> -Li Ching Yuen (1677-1933)

Stress occurs when anything important happens to you. There are acute physical stressors that trigger *fight or flight*, and chronic physical stressors that trigger a cascade of fuel partitioning. There are also psychological and social stressors such as relationships, debt, divorce, etc. Historically, mankind was faced with two major stressors: 1) starvation; and 2) lions and tigers and bears.

When encountered by a physiological stressor, the brain sends out a host of signals designed to prepare the body. *Fight or flight!,* for example, causes a rapid response via catecholamines (e.g., epinephrine) and a prolonged response mediated by cortisol. In response to a stressor, the hypothalamus secretes corticotrophin-releasing hormone (CRH), which stimulates the anterior pituitary to secrete adrenocorticotrophic hormone (ACTH), which stimulates the adrenals to secrete glucocorticoids (cortisol). Collectively, this is known as the hypothalamic-pituitary-adrenal, or HPA, axis:

Hypoth.	Ant. Pit.	adrenals
CRH →	ACTH →	Cortisol

Cortisol surges into the bloodstream, liberating fatty acids from adipose tissue and amino acids from muscle. Cortisol is in charge of making sure the right tissues are getting fuel in matters of life or death. During starvation, cortisol provides glucose for the brain; during *fight or flight*, cortisol provides fuel for skeletal muscle.

During the stress response, energy is diverted away from non-urgent functions. For example, free fatty acids and glucose are diverted away from adipose during starvation. During *fight of flight,* fuel is diverted away from the immune system, bone, etc. In times of starvation, food is not available (by definition), which creates a negative energy balance. Physical activity is markedly increased by *fight or flight*, which also creates a negative energy balance. In other words, the entire stress response system is specialized to operate in a state of negative energy balance. Things are very different today. Nowadays, we are well-fed and stressed out.

The physiological manifestations of chronic stress are of longer duration and lesser magnitude than those of acute stress. Cortisol, a major mediator in the acute stress response, is not markedly elevated in chronic stress compared to acute stress, but instead is 'out of balance.'

Dysregulated cortisol is bad news. It causes muscle wasting and visceral fat accumulation. Muscle wasting has devastating effects on energy balance, body composition, and quality of life. And in combination with "comfort foods," is a recipe for disaster.

Comfort foods

The craving for comfort foods in times of stress is like a cruel joke on mankind. Comfort foods help to *cope* with stress, not cure it. Historically, comfort foods and the stress response never coincided. There were rarely few situations when we would have to *fight or flight* while simultaneously enjoying some chocolate chip cookies or a potato casserole. Cortisol increases fuel availability in the bloodstream; so does eating. Combining the two causes an excess of fuel in the bloodstream[16], and since there are no tigers chasing us we don't need all of that fuel.

Cortisol stimulates the breakdown of triacylglycerols (fats) in adipose tissue, resulting in elevated plasma free fatty acids. Free fatty acids displace glucose oxidation in muscle, which preserves glucose for the brain. Cortisol also

---

[16] Unlike adipose tissue triacylglycerols or muscle glycogen, the bloodstream is *not* a buffer for excess calories.

causes skeletal muscle protein degradation, releasing amino acids into the bloodstream which are eventually converted into glucose for the brain during starvation or for muscle during *fight of flight.* However, when well-fed, stressed out, and sedentary, these fuels accumulate. When carb-rich comfort foods are added into the mix, insulin goes to work. Cortisol-induced lipolysis combined with insulin-induced fat storage leads to remodeling of adipose tissue storage depots. Fat storage increases in the viscera, contributing to the notorious beer belly. The visceral depot is one of the worst places to store fat; fat stored in subcutaneous depots like the hips and thighs may be unsightly, but is relatively benign. Visceral fat, on the other hand, is strongly associated with insulin resistance. Moreover, chronic low-grade stress combined with hyperinsulinemia ultimately favors net fat storage. The positive energy balance caused by overconsumption of carb-rich comfort foods further promotes hyperinsulinemia and the accumulation of fat mass.

Many of the interactions between the psychology and physiology of comfort foods have been worked out in animal models. In rats, for example, scientists have learned that sugar (sucrose)-containing beverages produce a significant "stress-dampening" effect. Ulrich-Lai and colleagues showed that sucrose actually attenuated the ACTH and behavioral responses to stress in rats, and this could actually be mimicked by saccharin (Ulrich-Lai, Ostrander et al. 2010). Interestingly, administering the sucrose (or saccharin) directly into their stomachs, bypassing the mouth, had no effect. The authors concluded that sucrose dampens the stress response not because of its calories but because of its sweet flavor.

Back to cortisol. Optimally, we would like insulin to act only on muscle and cortisol to act only on fat tissue. Insulin builds muscle and cortisol breaks down fat tissue. However, insulin also builds fat tissue and cortisol also breaks down muscle. Thus, these two hormones have an unfavorable effect on body composition.

Cortisol

Cortisol causes insulin resistance and visceral obesity. Cortisol-like drugs (corticosteroids, e.g., prednisone) are used to treat a variety of inflammatory conditions. To a patient with rheumatoid arthritis or bursitis, glucocorticoids can provide unmatched pain relief.

The side effects, as will be discussed below, are unpleasant, but living in pain is oftentimes much worse. Long-term side effects include weight-gain, visceral fat accumulation, loss of bone mass, and muscle wasting.

Cortisol directly causes peripheral insulin resistance. It reduces insulin-stimulated glucose uptake in muscles. After a carb-rich meal, this leads to hyperglycemia. Cortisol inhibits insulin's anti-lipolytic effects on adipose which contributes to postprandial hyperlipidemia and the elevated free fatty acids further antagonize glucose utilization. Cortisol causes protein degradation in skeletal muscle which releases amino acids that are converted to glucose by the liver. During starvation, those free fatty acids would be utilized primarily by muscle and the glucose would be preserved for the brain. Unfortunately, this system is evolutionarily outdated as we are no longer subject to periods of starvation or life and death *fight or flight* situations.

An interesting experiment was performed to determine the relationship between the magnitude of an individual's response to stress and how efficiently their body accumulates fat mass. This study was done with rams (non-castrated male sheep), and although humans are quite different from sheep, many hormonal effects are similar among mammals (Knott, Cummins et al. 2010). In this study the stressor was actually artificial: an ACTH injection. In general, the stress begins in the brain with the secretion of CRH from the hypothalamus which causes ACTH secretion from the anterior pituitary:

Hypoth.	Ant. Pit.	adrenals
CRH →	ACTH →	Cortisol

Then the ACTH stimulates the adrenals to secrete cortisol which comprises a large part of the stress response. However, for a more consistent biological response, and to isolate the cortisol response, researchers just skipped right to injecting ACTH and measuring the increase in cortisol.

After ACTH injections ($2\mu g/kg$), the researchers measured cortisol levels and divided the rams into low and high responders. Baseline cortisol was 67 nM and increased to 113 nM in low responders and to 216 nM in high responders. That is quite a big difference in a seemingly homogeneous population of rams. All the rams weighed ~55 kg and had a body fat level of ~12% at baseline. Then the researchers did nothing but measure food intake for the next two months. By the end of the study, all of the rams put on about 13 kg (this study took place during a major growth phase for the rams, like puberty for humans). Body fat in the low responders increased by 1% and was <u>three times greater in the high responders</u>. Importantly, all the rams gained approximately the same amount of body weight so they were apparently in equally positive energy balance. This suggests that being a high responder, someone who is easily stressed out, causes a negative nutrient partitioning effect whereby weight gain is comprised of less muscle and more fat compared to less stressed out individuals. In this study, this difference was entirely due to the initial screening of cortisol responsivity.

One interesting caveat was that high responders ate more than low responders. They gained the same amount of weight, so this means that energy expenditure must have been higher in high responders than low responders. In other words, simply being a high responder caused some of the excess energy intake to be selectively invested into fat tissue. If you are a low responder, this could possibly be interpreted to mean that if you happen to overeat, there is a smaller chance of it increasing fat mass compared to someone who is stressed out. **Furthermore, the hormonal milieu, cortisol responsivity in this case, can impact nutrient partitioning. The amount of fat that is stored, even when in energy balance, is not a simple matter of calories.**

Those findings were confirmed in a similar model but completely different experimental paradigm. In this study (Lee, Giles et al. 2005), sheep were immunized against ACTH. In other words, the immune system would attack and degrade much of the secreted ACTH before it had a chance to stimulate cortisol secretion. These sheep thus had an artificially lower stress response, much like Knott's 'low responders.'

Next, the researchers induced a stressful situation by disrupting the sheep's natural social hierarchy. They found that, despite all the sheep experiencing the exact same psychologically stressful situation, those who had a lower biological stress response accumulated significantly less fat mass over time.

Cortisol isn't the only mediator of the stress response with relevance to energy balance, but it is a good example of how body weight, and more importantly fat mass, is not a matter determined exclusively by calories. Different macronutrients, hormones, and stress are all capable of contributing to the determination of how much fat mass that is lost or gained *within energy balance*.

Stress and diet
Chill out! Resolving the underlying stressor is the only cure, per se. Stress seems to direct the energy from ingested food into fat tissue, which is compounded if those foods are insulinogenic (comfort foods). If you absolutely need to eat in times of stress, avoid the standard carb-rich comfort foods and prepare a proper low-glycemic meal. Perhaps focusing on cooking will take your mind off the stress. Go for some green leafy or cruciferous veggies to replete your vitamins and minerals. The protein from a hearty cut of meat will help to counteract the cortisol-induced skeletal muscle degradation, and the fat will help convince your brain that you're not really hungry. Alternatively, a fatty fish like salmon would provide the protein as well as fish oils which promote well-being and can lessen depressive and anxiety symptoms. A healthy diet can attenuate many of the worst symptoms of stress.

Visceral fat

As stated above, subcutaneous adipose tissue occurs just beneath the skin while visceral adipose is found within the peritoneum, or around the intestines. Excess subcutaneous fat produces the "pear" figure while excess visceral fat produces the "apple." While it may be more unsightly, subcutaneous adipose tissue is relatively benign. It is a safe place to store fat.

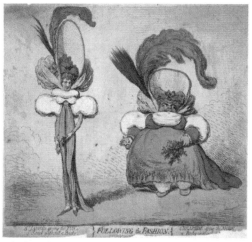

On the right, the "apple" figure. The woman on the left is just plain thin.

The body is not meant to store fat within the viscera. Visceral adipose tissue is an example of an ectopic fat depot. That is, fat is not normally stored there, but certain conditions such as stress or hyperinsulinemia create an unnatural environment that results in visceral fat deposition. Other examples of ectopic fat depots are the liver, as occurs during high carb or fructose feeding, and in muscle, as occurs in obesity. Endurance athletes also accumulate intramuscular lipids but this isn't necessarily ectopic because it is functional; the fat is used as a source of fuel for aerobic exercise.

Visceral fat is actually more strongly associated with morbidities and overall mortality than body weight. And as stated above, the decision to store fat in the viscera as opposed to subcutaneously is not specifically dictated by energy balance but by the hormonal milieu. And it is never a good thing. Alternatively, subcutaneous fat is relatively benign. Some data in support of this comes from studies of liposuction patients. In a study by Klein and colleagues, a battery of health parameters were analyzed before and 3 months after surgical removal of a significant quantity of their subcutaneous adipose tissue (Klein, Fontana et al. 2004). The patients weighed between 200 and 250 pounds, and 20 pounds of subcutaneous fat was surgically removed during the procedure. Accordingly, they weighed around 20 pounds less after surgery. They were given no dietary instructions. Removal of subcutaneous fat resulted in no change in plasma glucose, insulin, or markers of inflammation. Insulin sensitivity was completely unaffected. Leptin levels declined, as expected because in general leptin levels reflect total body fat. If subcutaneous fat was detrimental, then its removal should have benefitted these patients. But there was no effect. Subcutaneous adipose is harmless and its removal is purely aesthetic.

Another way to view these findings is to focus on the fact that these patients lost 20 pounds of fat but didn't get healthier. If they had lost that much weight by diet, there would have definitely been marked improvements in glucose metabolism and insulin sensitivity. I would even go so far as to say that if they had lost only 10 pounds of fat by dieting, their health would have improved measurably. Thus, dieting is a more important variable than adiposity, per se, in determining health outcomes.

Subcutaneous adipose tissue is more insulin sensitive than visceral, and visceral adipose tissue is more prone to lipolysis. Collectively, these two observations confirm that the body is not supposed to store fat in the viscera, but unnatural conditions such as chronic stress or hyperinsulinemia alter the metabolic landscape and favor ectopic fat storage.

The human liposuction data are sufficient to exonerate subcutaneous adipose, although such evidence implicating visceral fat is less direct. For this, we must consider animal studies. Borst studied the impact of visceral fat removal in rats (Borst, Conover et al. 2005). Not surprisingly, within just a few weeks of surgery almost every parameter of glucose metabolism and insulin sensitivity showed marked improvements. This has since been confirmed in both mice and rats. Although liposuction generally only targets the unsightly subcutaneous fat, surgical removal of visceral fat for the treatment of metabolic diseases is probably not far off.

Interestingly, Gabriely and colleagues showed that visceral fat removal in rats was comparable to calorie restriction in improving glucose metabolism and insulin sensitivity (Gabriely, Ma et al. 2002)! Since visceral fat is naturally reduced during calorie restriction, it is possible that less visceral fat should be considered a candidate to explain the mechanism of how calorie restriction improves health outcomes.

One final piece of evidence confirming the safety and harm of subcutaneous and visceral fat, respectively, comes from the pharmaceutical industry. Thiazolidinediones (TZDs) are prescribed to type II diabetics to lower blood glucose and improve insulin sensitivity. The major drawback is that type II diabetics are usually obese and TZDs cause weight gain. But they considerably improve health in these patients. How can this be? TZDs stimulate the expansion of subcutaneous fat, which causes weight gain, but is also draws fat out of all other ectopic storage sites like visceral adipose, liver, and skeletal muscle. In other words, TZDs redistribute fat storage from unhealthy places to the comparatively metabolically inert subcutaneous depot.

Chapter 11.
Diet and lifespan

The oldest currently living
organism known: a 4,800 year
old bristlecone pine in the White
Mountains of California, USA

Diet is the major *controllable* determinant of "healthspan," or duration of morbidity-free life. It can also affect various aspects of the aging process. There are some notable examples of how diet, and the major hormones that are regulated by diet, impact the aging process. A direct effect of diet on aging is observed during caloric restriction. Indirect evidence has been demonstrated in animal models with manipulations in leptin or insulin signaling.

Caloric Restriction

Caloric restriction is a dietary regimen that entails a reduction in overall calorie intake by anywhere from 15% to 50% percent relative to baseline. It has been promoted as a possible cure for aging and in many species this has held true. In rodents, for example, a 30% to 40% caloric restriction increases lifespan by almost half. And this is not just an increase in the senior years; the animals are leaner and significantly more robust for a greater portion of their life.

The most famous study of caloric restriction began in the 1980's on a group of rhesus monkeys (Ramsey, Colman et al. 2000). These animals were caloric restricted by 30% and were still going on strong at the time of this book. Caloric restricted monkeys have markedly less fat mass, and lower blood glucose and insulin levels similar to what is seen in rodents. The lower glucose levels may not simply be a passive effect of caloric restriction, however. It is possible that chronically low glucose levels are one of the mechanisms as to *how* caloric restriction improves health. High glucose is toxic to many tissues and can bind to and impair the function of a variety of proteins in a process known as glycation (Rahmadi, Steiner et al. 2011). At the cellular level, reduced exposure to glucose decreases cell damage, improves markers of the aging process, and enhances viability. Collectively, these findings suggest that glucose may have a critical role in the aging process and that maintaining healthy glucose levels may be an effective anti-aging strategy.

Additional support for the link between diet and aging comes from studies of genetically modified mice. Animals lacking one or more components of the insulin signaling pathways exhibit increased lifespan. The effects produced by genetically impairing insulin signaling are similar to carbohydrate restriction. This connection links lowered blood glucose levels *and* insulin directly to caloric restriction. In other words, it is possible that some of the effects of caloric restriction can be mimicked by selectively restricting carbohydrates.

Resveratrol

In vino veritas! Resveratrol is a compound that naturally occurs in the skin of grapes and is concentrated in red wine. It is thought to be synthesized during times of stress (drought, high winds, etc.) to function as a protective agent. Grapes grown in exactly those conditions tend to produce superior wines, so a perk to drinking fine wine is that you may be getting more resveratrol. Why is this good? Some of the benefits of caloric restriction seem to be related to a reduced metabolic rate. The flipside is that things which increase metabolic rate should have an opposite, pro-aging effect. Unfortunately this includes a LOT of activities; sports, eating, and reproduction just to name a few. Resveratrol appears to mimic the effects of calorie restriction without the need for actually reducing energy expenditure. In other words, with resveratrol, you could theoretically reap some of the benefits of caloric restriction while eating cake… OK, that may not be entirely true, but resveratrol certainly does appear to be very close to a miracle drug.

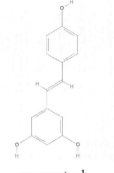

resveratrol

Caloric restriction creates an absolute energy deficit at the cellular level. This stimulates the activity of protective enzymes known as sirtuins. Sirtuins are generally considered the master biological mediators of aging. There is a very strong inverse correlation between the biological response to caloric restriction and the aging process.

During energy deficit, sirtuins exhibit a variety of tissue-specific effects. For example, during caloric restriction the body needs to switch to burning fat for fuel in order to preserve glucose for the brain. Therefore, sirtuins help mobilize fatty acids from adipose tissue. In the liver, sirtuins stimulate fatty acid oxidation which creates ketones. Ketones are used as fuel by a variety of tissues, which decreases their use of glucose (further preserving glucose for the brain). This also stimulates gluconeogenesis (yet again, to provide glucose for the brain). All of these functions are part of the response to fasting or caloric restriction and all are important for survival. More importantly, this set of responses is actually *healthier* than the status quo, and this is where resveratrol comes in[17].

Resveratrol activates sirtuins just like caloric restriction. While the effects on lifespan are less robust than caloric restriction, many of the benefits of resveratrol are similar. In one landmark study, resveratrol was put to the test and performed amazingly (Baur, Pearson et al. 2006). In this study the researchers fed one group of mice standard chow and another group a high-calorie diet that is well-known to induce obesity in mice. Half of the obese animals were then treated with resveratrol.

Resveratrol did not affect food intake or body weight. By itself, this result suggests that energy balance was clearly maintained. In other words, resveratrol had no effect on nutrient

---

[17] General disclaimer: while the biologic and metabolic improvements associated with resveratrol supplementation are well-documented, the exact mechanism of action is unknown.

partitioning effects in this model. The most profound findings were on lifespan. By around 29 months of age, 42% of the mice fed standard chow died (of natural causes). At this time point, 58% of the obese mice passed away. And only 48% of the obese mice given resveratrol had died suggesting that resveratrol almost completely negated the effects of obesity on lifespan.

Fat mass is thought to be a negative regulator of lifespan, and it correlates well in certain animal models. Energy expenditure is also thought to negatively regulate lifespan. Resveratrol-treated obese mice had significantly more fat mass than the chow group but lived just as long, dissociating the connection between fat mass and lifespan. The resveratrol-treated obese mice had the same energy expenditure as the control obese mice but they lived significantly longer, dissociating the connection between energy expenditure and lifespan. Thus, resveratrol debunked both theories of aging. However, resveratrol treatment significantly lowered glucose and insulin levels down to those seen in the lean, chow-fed animals. Therefore, in this model, glucose and insulin levels, not energy expenditure or fat mass, correlated with lifespan.

Besides implicating blood levels of glucose and insulin in the aging process, what does this mean for us? Unfortunately, there is only about 1 mg of resveratrol in a glass of red wine. The mice were fed 22 mg/kg, which would be 1,680 mg for someone weighing 165 pounds. So no, it is impossible to drink nearly enough red wine. Although it may be considerably less than what the mathematical dose escalation would suggest. For example, it is possible that, milligram for milligram, resveratrol in wine is more potent than isolated resveratrol. Wine may contain other compounds that increase the stability and enhance the bioavailability of resveratrol. The alcohol in wine may act synergistically with resveratrol.   In sum, although I am a great enthusiast of red wine, the benefits of resveratrol would be better sought through a nutritional supplement or pharmaceutical drug. Indeed, there is a great interest in developing a clinically relevant analog to resveratrol among the big pharmaceutical companies.

But to get back to the main point, the example of resveratrol shows that blood **glucose and insulin**, not fat mass and energy expenditure, are directly related to lifespan.

Leptin-deficiency

Mice lacking leptin are "genetically obese." Actually, they are enormous. It is absurd. *And* their lifespan is considerably reduced (Harrison, Archer et al. 1984). In a profound study by Harrison and colleagues (1984), the normal mouse lifespan was shown to be almost 33 months. A 33% reduction in caloric intake extended this by approximately 23% to 43 months. Body fat was 22% (~7 grams) in normal mice and reduced by 40% down to 13% (~3 grams) in caloric restricted mice.

Normal mice:
- 33% calories → -40% fat mass → + 32% lifespan.

Leptin-deficient mice ate a third more, weighed twice as much, and had three times the fat mass of normal mice. Their lifespan was 10% shorter, approximately 30 months. Caloric restricted leptin-deficient mice still carried twice as much a fat mass as non-restricted normal mice but lived for almost 44 months! In other words, the extension in lifespan was due specifically to calorie restriction per se, not reduced fat mass.

Leptin-deficient mice:

-52% calories → - 28% fat mass → + 46% lifespan

Let me get this straight: the leptin-deficient mice were *more* caloric restricted but lost *less* fat, and had a *greater* life extension. Huh? Leptin signals "well-fed" status to the brain. In leptin deficiency, the brain thinks it is starving so metabolic rate is considerably reduced to preserve energy. This is why leptin deficient mice lost less fat mass and may be one of the reasons why weight loss is easy at first (high leptin levels → high metabolic rate) but becomes more difficult over time (weight loss → lower fat mass → lower leptin levels → brain thinks it is starving → lower metabolic rate).

One caveat to this study was that the leptin-deficient mice were more severely calorie restricted than the normal mice. The researchers wanted to feed both groups of mice the same amount of food during the restriction phase of the study, and since leptin-deficient mice ate more to begin with (4.2 grams vs. 3 grams per day), they were more severely restricted (both groups were given 2 grams of food per day during calorie restriction). Although this may complicate interpreting the results, one thing is clear: the caloric restriction per se, not fat mass, dictated longevity in this study. Furthermore, this lends support to the theory that although both are reduced by caloric restriction, **metabolic rate** but not fat mass is the major driver of longevity.

The general conclusions of the Harrison study were confirmed in rats. Rats harboring a natural mutation in the leptin gene are known as Zucker fatty rats. In a study by Johnson and colleagues (Johnson, Stern et al. 1997), 3 groups of rats were studies. One lean control group fed ad libitum, one group of obese Zucker fatty rats fed ad libitum, and one group of Zuckers who were pair-fed to the lean controls. Zuckers eat more than lean rats and are much fatter. Food intake is only modestly increased, but the difference in energy balance is magnified because Zuckers lack leptin, so they naturally have a lower metabolic rate. The pair-fed Zuckers ate just as much as control (that is, by definition, pair-feeding) but weighed significantly more (because of their lower metabolic rate). Lean rats lived for 36 months, on average, and obesity reduced this by 25% to 27 months. Pair-feeding increased Zucker's lifespan by 22% to 34 months, almost completely negating the effect of obesity on lifespan.

	food intake (g/week)	BW (g)	Fat mass		lifespan (months)
			g	%	
lean control	120	298	34	10%	36
obese	130	485	201	41%	27
pair-fed	120	407	177	42%	34

The pair-fed Zucker rats weighed significantly less than obese rats, although both groups had approximately 40% body fat. The pair-fed rats had a lower metabolic rate (they ate less and weighed less) so they lived significantly longer.

The pair-fed Zuckers weighed more and had significantly more fat mass than the lean controls. They were eating just as much which suggests a markedly slower metabolic rate, and they almost lived as long as the lean controls. According to their metabolic rate, the obese rats should have lived longer. However, fat mass is a negative regulator of lifespan, so in this case it would appear as though the longevity benefits of a lower metabolic rate were nullified by elevated **fat mass**.

Metabolic rate and lifespan

There is substantial evidence that metabolic rate is closely linked to lifespan. Lifespan may be limited by the total amount of energy expended. In other words, we die when a certain amount of calories are burned. An average person may expend 100 million kilocalories in their life:

3,425 kilocalories per day
X 29,200 days (80 years)
100,000,000 kilocalories

Perhaps there is a limit?
-Calorie restriction is thought to extend lifespan by reducing metabolic rate.

-Cold-blooded animals have markedly lower metabolic rates because they expend much less energy on maintaining their body temperature (which is oftentimes simply a few degrees above the ambient temperature, whatever that may be). Cold-blooded animals live longer than similar-sized species of warm-blooded animals, and their lifespan is further lengthened in colder climates.

-Flying burns way more calories than walking, thus flies have a much greater total energy expenditure, relatively, because that is how they get around. Flies that can't fly live substantially longer.

-Mice and bats are similarly sized and warm-blooded but bats can live almost 10 times longer. At first, this appears contradictory; however, bats spend much more time resting and frequently reduce their metabolic rate for extended periods of time (torpor, hibernation).

There are some notable contradictory examples that cannot be so easily explained.

-Worker bees live only a few months but the queen can live for over 5 years. Furthermore, she just sits around eating excessively for her entire life! AND she is constantly reproducing! Although workers fly more than the queen, it is unlikely that the increased energy expended during flight is enough to match the queen. The total lifelong energy expenditure is markedly greater for the queen, and she lives longer. It's good to be the queen.

-FIRKO mice...

FIRKO mice

As discussed above, to optimize the efficacy of insulin on nutrient partitioning would require enhanced insulin sensitivity in muscle tissue but insulin resistance selectively in fat tissue. This would allow for the anabolic effects of insulin on muscle growth but inhibit the anabolic effects of insulin on fat storage. A line of mice lacking the insulin receptor selectively in fat tissue was created to study the metabolic effects of such a scenario (Bluher, Michael et al. 2002). They are known as the FIRKO mice; Fat-specific insulin receptor knockout. Mice lacking insulin signaling in fat tissue (FIRKO) is comparable to fat-specific insulin resistance (aka nutrient partitioning).

For starters, as predicted from what we know about the obesogenic effects of insulin, FIRKO mice were healthy, carried about 60% less body fat than normal mice, and were 20% lighter (Bluher, Kahn et al. 2003). Interestingly, they ate the same amount of food as normal mice. Given that they weigh 20% less, this suggests that their total energy expenditure must be markedly higher.

some digressions

-If they weighed less and ate less, their energy expenditure would be lower than normal mice, but the same *per unit of body weight*.

-If they weighed less but ate more, their energy expenditure would be higher, and much much higher p*er unit of body weight*.

-In this case, however, FIRKO weighed less but ate the same amount as normal mice. Therefore, energy expenditure is unchanged in FIRKO mice, but increased *per unit of body weight*.

This also means that they ate more *per unit of body weight*. In keeping with the laws of energy balance, this means that FIRKO mice were more physically active or had a higher energy expenditure. Alternatively, it is possible that the dynamics of the fat tissue were *fundamentally* altered to store less fat. Ummm, well, can I say that? Actually, the fat tissue was *genetically* altered to lack insulin signaling; so yes, perhaps fat-specific insulin resistance fundamentally alters fat tissue dynamics. In other words, FIRKO mice could have less fat mass but the same level of energy expenditure. As described ad nauseum in previous chapters, increased fat mass is associated with an energy surplus and the opposite should also be true: decreased fat mass associated with an energy deficit. However, at least in the case of the FIRKO mice, it would appear that the laws of energy balance may have been maintained in a relatively straightforward manner... except for the fact that energy expenditure was not measured. At this point, we can only assume that lower body weight despite normal food intake means increased energy expenditure.

These mice appeared healthier than normal, so the researchers went straight to the one of the biggest questions in the field: what about their lifespan? In accord with previous research, they found that about half of the normal mice were still alive by 30 months of age. Interestingly, roughly 80% of FIRKO mice were still alive by that age, and mean lifespan was increased by 18% to 34 months. Maximal lifespan was 41 months, almost as high as leptin-deficient caloric restricted mice. However, increased lifespan in caloric restriction was attributed to reduced energy expenditure, and specifically *not* to reduced fat mass. Leptin-deficient caloric restricted mice have *more* fat mass than normal mice but live longer due to a lower metabolic rate. FIRKO mice have a higher metabolic rate but live longer due to lower fat mass? Resveratrol-treated mice have more fat mass *and* normal metabolic rate but live longer!? Well, which is it? Can you have both? All three models have one thing in common ... [*dramatic pause*]   lower glucose and insulin levels.

FOXO3a

Human studies on aging are rare, but examining DNA polymorphisms has allowed investigators to ask if there is a genetic component to longevity. DNA polymorphisms are short regions of DNA that are different between different groups of people. They are similar within a family, thus you and your parents and siblings likely have the same polymorphisms. Researchers compare hundreds of DNA polymorphisms with health outcomes in thousands of people and look for correlations.

The Hawaii Lifespan Study has been going on since the 1960's and includes primarily Japanese-American men living in Hawaii (Willcox, Donlon et al. 2008). In this study, the researchers compared health records and DNA samples of men who lived for at least 95 years ("longevity" cases) to those who died before the age of 81 ("average-lived" control group). They were looking for DNA polymorphisms that were significantly more or less abundant in the longevity cases compared to control. They found that significantly more longevity cases had a polymorphism in a gene known as FOXO3a, suggesting FOXO3a may regulate longevity. They then looked at younger men who were still alive and found that those with the FOXO3a polymorphism were significantly *healthier* than controls. Thus, FOXO3a might play a role in lifespan *and healthspan*. Lastly, they found that *anyone* with the polymorphism had significantly lower insulin levels and higher insulin sensitivity. Basically, having the FOXO3a polymorphism made them healthier and tripled their chances of living to 100. Is it plausible to assume that the polymorphism *caused* the health and longevity outcomes? I believe so, because people with the polymorphism had increased insulin sensitivity and lower insulin levels. They were leaner. We know that these factors are protective against diseases, and accordingly, those men were healthier. It is not proof, but the data are consistent, logical, and quite good.

These findings were confirmed in a German population (Flachsbart, Caliebe et al. 2009). In this study, over one thousand unrelated Germans were recruited. The "longevity group" was between 95 and 105 years old and the controls were in their 60's. They also included a population of more than 500 French people to ensure adequate genetic diversity. In accord with the data from Japanese-Americans living in Hawaii, the FOXO3a polymorphism was associated with increased longevity in both the German and French populations. This has been confirmed in Italians (Anselmi, Malovini et al. 2009), Ashkenazi Jews, Californians, New Englanders (Pawlikowska, Hu et al. 2009), and Chinese (Li, Wang et al. 2009) populations.

Why is all this relevant? What does FOXO3a have to do with poor, misunderstood calories? As alluded to in the Willcox study on longevity in Japanese-American Hawaiians, FOXO3a is involved in mediating the effects of insulin. Actually, FOXO3a is activated in the fasting state (think: caloric restriction); glucose ingestion and the subsequent hyperinsulinemia inactivates FOXO3a. Reduced insulin levels would result in more active FOXO3a. Caloric restriction lowers insulin, glucose, fat mass, metabolic rate, and increases longevity. Resveratrol lowers insulin, glucose, and increases longevity despite no change in fat mass or metabolic rate. Caloric restriction lowers insulin and glucose levels in leptin-deficient mice and enhances longevity despite elevated fat mass. Deletion of the insulin receptor in fat tissue reduces insulin and glucose and increases longevity despite having an elevated metabolic rate. Neither fat mass nor metabolic rate can completely explain the longevity phenotype all of in these models. The one thing they all have in common is lower insulin and glucose levels than their shorter-lived controls. Due to low insulin and glucose levels, the activity of FOXO3a is expected to be high in each model, and a FOXO3a polymorphism in humans is associated with longevity. The most proximal causal factor is insulin and glucose, and by extension dietary carbohydrates.

Does this refer only high glycemic index carbohydrates and sugar, or does it apply to all carbohydrates? The United Kingdom Prospective Diabetes Study began in 1977 and was designed to determine if intensive glucose control was superior to conventional therapy (diet) in type II diabetes. Intensive glucose control consisted of insulin, sulfonylureas, or metformin. Sulfonylureas increase glucose-induced insulin secretion. Metformin decreases liver glucose production and increases insulin sensitivity. So these patients basically kept their carbohydrate intake constant but had lower blood glucose levels because of the drug treatments. As expected, elevated insulin levels (the result of sulfonylureas and insulin injections), caused weight gain. But importantly, mortality was not reduced by intensive glucose control.

The same thing was shown in the ACCORD study, which compared conventional with intensive glucose lowering therapy in diabetic patients (Gerstein, Miller et al. 2008). This study included over 10,000 subjects and was stopped prematurely because mortality was significantly higher in the intensive group. Weight gain was also a prominent side effect of intensive therapy.

Type II diabetes and high blood glucose reduce lifespan. In the Balkau study, risk for all-cause mortality increased linearly with increased blood glucose (Balkau, Shipley et al. 1998). The United Kingdom Prospective Diabetes Study showed that keeping glucose levels low *by intensive drug therapy* does not improve longevity. Collectively, these findings suggest that *how glucose is kept low* matters. Glucose levels must be kept low by *decreasing the influx of glucose*. There is one clear way to do this: decrease the total intake of carbohydrates. The United Kingdom Prospective Diabetes Study demonstrated that simply lowering blood glucose levels doesn't work. The preponderance of evidence suggests that carbohydrate restriction is the optimal way to reduce glycemia. Moreover, increased insulin is associated with reduced longevity in each of the abovementioned animal models, the United Kingdom Prospective Diabetes Study, and the FOXO3a polymorphism studies. I see a pattern.

Cancer

Tumor cells consume glucose as their primary fuel. In some studies that look at glycemia, insulin treatment, and mortality, no effect on mortality is observed. One reason for this might be due to the nature of the therapeutic intervention. Two mechanisms by which intensive drug therapy lowers blood glucose are: 1) drugs that stimulate insulin secretion (sulfonylureas); and 2) insulin injections. Both result in higher insulin, lower glucose, and weight gain. One possible explanation for not seeing a major effect on mortality is that any benefits of lower glucose levels are offset by the detriment of increased weight gain. Another possibility is that elevated insulin levels directly increase mortality.

Knatterud designed a study to look at mortality in diabetics treated conventionally (diet) or with one of two different insulin regimens (Knatterud, Klimt et al. 1978). As expected, glycaemia was markedly reduced by insulin therapy. However, mortality was similar in all three groups. A breakdown of the causes of mortality showed that most deaths in the conventionally treated group were cancer-related. Interestingly, most deaths in the insulin-treated groups were due to cardiovascular causes such as heart attack or sudden cardiac death. The blood glucose levels were markedly higher in the conventionally treated group, and glucose is the preferred fuel for growing tumor cells(Warburg, Wind et al. 1927).

Therefore it is possible that subjects in the conventionally treated group had more cancer-related deaths *because* of their chronically elevated blood glucose levels. By lowering glucose with insulin injections, the other two groups reduced the glucose available for tumor growth but were then exposed to chronically high levels of insulin. Does insulin promote cardiovascular mortality? Is insulin atherogenic? These questions are important because if the answer is yes, then the use of drug therapy to control blood glucose levels needs to be seriously reconsidered.

Chapter 12.
Get fatter without a positive energy balance

`

When calories are restricted, a certain set of biological phenomena are expected to occur in order to sustain energy balance. In general, if food intake declines, either body weight or energy expenditure must also decline to maintain energy balance. Although people do indeed lose weight on calorie restricted diets, a major benefit [on lifespan] is thought to come from the reduced metabolic rate. An elevated metabolic rate means that your body is burning a lot of fuel. A byproduct of this is increased production of free radicals, which literally *cause* aging.

Energy balance is always maintained. Theoretically, body weight could remain constant during calorie restriction if energy expenditure declined to match the new lower level of food intake. This often occurs when people suddenly become bedridden, although the cause and effect are reversed. In this case, energy expenditure is reduced which decreases appetite. Unfortunately, however, most deviations like these produce unfavorable outcomes. Although reduced food intake might sustain a constant body weight in somebody who is suddenly bedridden, they are likely to gain fat mass and lose muscle. This is primarily due to the "use it or lose it" principle of skeletal muscle. That is, muscle tissue undergoes "disuse atrophy" during extended periods of rest.

Herein lays an interesting paradigm. Bedridden status reduces energy expenditure, which is matched by reduced energy intake, but fat mass increases.   In other words, fat tissue can grow despite no change in energy balance. To be clear, this suggests that **you can get fatter *without* a positive energy balance**.

This was also been observed in a recent animal study (Li, Cope et al. 2010). In this study, one group of mice were fed a 5% calorie restricted diet and followed for 3-4 weeks. Two variations of calorie restriction were performed: in the first, caloric intake was measured in the beginning of the study to be around 10 kilocalories. Then for the rest of the study, the mice were fed 9.5 kilocalories. So they were eating <u>5% less than baseline</u>. The other variation tracked the calorie intake of a control group of mice and constantly adjusted the amount of food given to the calorie restricted group so that they were always eating <u>5% less than the control group</u>. Although it was clever of the researchers to include both variations, the results were the same. There were many findings that, if viewed in isolation, would suggest that the laws of energy balance were violated. For starters, despite eating less, the mice didn't weigh less. OK, this could only be possible if, for example, some other aspect of energy expenditure was reduced to match the reduced food intake. So the researchers measured physical activity. Much to their dismay, it was unchanged, and actually increased at certain time points! In other words, the mice were eating less and moving more and not losing any weight. To make a long story short, their total metabolic rate was indeed reduced, energy balance was maintained, and everyone could sleep easy that night. There was one finding, however, that was so surprising that the researchers actually repeated the entire study. The calorie restricted mice lost lean mass and put on fat mass. In other words, **the mice got fatter without a positive energy balance**.

How could this happen? For starters, lean mass (muscle) was lost. This might be explained by the reduction in food intake. Muscle is the major contributor to energy expenditure. If food intake declines, and muscle is lost in order to reduce energy expenditure, energy balance could be maintained. The only strange part of that conclusion is that it implies that muscle was lost *in order to* reduce energy expenditure. Why would muscle do this? Perhaps it is a novel variation of the "use it or lose it" principle.

When calorie intake is reduced, leptin levels decline rapidly signaling "starvation" mode to the brain. This decreases energy expenditure in order to preserve energy stores. Previously, the decline in energy expenditure would have been predicted to occur by decreased physical activity. And reduced physical activity could cause muscle loss due to "use it or lose it." But physical activity was unchanged. Therefore, it is possible that the decline in metabolic rate was manifested in processes other than physical activity *in muscle tissue*. This means that "use it or lose it" could apply to activities ("using it") that occur at rest. Clearly, this is a marked deviation from the energy balance dogma. And it has kept me up at nights.

What processes could these be? None were measured or even suggested by the authors of the study, but I suppose it could possibly be reduced activity of ion channels, or possibly reduced futile cycling. More research is severely warranted.

So muscle was lost *in order to* balance the reduced food intake. Where did the energy come from to build fat mass? This may have already been explained... if metabolic rate was reduced down to match food intake, energy balance would be maintained. If metabolic rate was reduced even further, it would produce a *relative* energy surplus. Perhaps this is precisely what occurred to these mice. Thus, muscle was lost *in order to* balance the reduced food intake, and metabolic rate declined *in order to* create a relative positive energy balance selectively in the fat tissue. Why would something like this occur? It is very strange, to be sure, but may have had something to do with the stress of the feeding regimen. The body thinks it is starving, so preserving fat mass becomes a priority. Maybe the systems that work to preserve fat mass during starvation are the same as those that build fat mass during energy surplus. For now, however, trying to explain these observations without defying the laws of energy balance has caused gray hairs to appear in my beard. A positive energy balance selectively in the fat tissue? ...

Gray hairs set aside for the moment, the mice got fatter without a positive energy balance. Can this happen to us? (does it matter *how*?) These results suggest that fat tissue has a propensity to grow regardless of energy balance. In the abovementioned study, the trigger may have been the hormonal response to a stressful feeding regimen. Type I diabetics are usually very thin but develop fat deposits around their insulin injection sites (Griffin, Feder et al. 2001); thus, in type I diabetics, the trigger is insulin. In both situations, **fat mass grew because of the hormonal milieu, not an energy surplus *per se*.**

Lose more fat sans more negative energy balance

Larson-Meyer and colleagues performed a study that compared different types of energy deficit on body composition (Larson-Meyer, Heilbronn et al. 2006). This study is interesting because it clarified an important principle of **The poor, misunderstood calorie**. They recruited a population of overweight subjects and assigned them to one of three different calorie reduced diets (and a weight-stable control). A strength of this study, right off the bat, is the inclusion of a weight-stable control group. People behave differently when they are being watched; there is a notable 'effect of the observer on the observed[18].' People's behaviors will change during the course of the study, independent of the experimental intervention, therefore by comparing any changes that occurred between baseline and the end of the study does not differentiate which changes were

---

[18] Margaret Mead

due to the intervention from those that were caused by participation in the study. Presumably, the behavior of people in the weight-stable control group will also change during the course of the study, so comparing subjects in an active treatment group to weight-stable controls is a way to isolate effects of the intervention from effects of study participation.

First, energy expenditure was measured by doubly-labeled water. This technique gives a decent approximation of energy expenditure *in free-living individuals*. In brief, subjects are instructed to drink a large quantity of doubly-labeled water; i.e., water "H_2O" where the hydrogen and oxygen are replaced by the stable isotopes deuterium and oxygen-18, respectively: "$D_2{}^{18}O$." The D_2 (stable isotope of hydrogen) is excreted as water D_2O (urine, sweat, etc.), while the ^{18}O is excreted as carbon dioxide $C^{18}O_2$ *and* water $H_2{}^{18}O$. D_2O and $H_2{}^{18}O$ are both physiologically the same and are excreted at the same rate. Excretion of $C^{18}O_2$ depends on how much carbon dioxide you are producing; higher energy expenditure means higher carbon dioxide production. Therefore the difference between D_2 and ^{18}O reflects a general approximation of energy expenditure. An advantage and flaw of this technique is that it takes the average energy expenditure over two weeks. That is an advantage because long-term energy balance is more important for body weight regulation in free-living individuals. It is a disadvantage because the technique cannot easily be used to determine which component of energy expenditure is changed, which is fortunately not our concern at this point.

After obtaining baseline energy expenditure values, each subject was assigned to one of four groups:

1) Weight-stable control

2) 25% energy deficit via diet alone

3) 12.5% energy deficit via diet +
    12.5% energy deficit via exercise

4) 15% weight loss via diet

Basically, group 2 was assigned a 25% calorie restricted standard low-fat diet, while group three were assigned a 12.5% calorie restriction and 12.5% additional calories spent during physical activity (walking, jogging, etc.). Group 4 consisted of an ultra-low calorie diet (890 kilocalories per day) until they lost 15% of their starting body weight, and then calories were tapered up to keep them stable at their reduced weight. This turned out to be similar to the 25% energy deficient groups (groups 2 and 3). This study would have been included in the nutrient partitioning chapter, although the exercise intervention (jogging) is not the type expected to sufficiently induce a state of nutrient partitioning, which would generally consist of high intensity anaerobic exercise.

They found that, indeed, a 25% energy deficit produced similar weight loss in both groups. But I thought you said exercise won't promote weight loss! 1) This study was only 6 months, not reflective of a long-term lifestyle change; and 2) exercise *alone* will not promote long-term weight loss because food intake often increases to compensate for the exercise-induced energy deficit. In this study, both groups were assigned a strict diet; so even if exercise *did* make the subjects in group 3 more hungry, they weren't permitted to eat more because they were on a strict diet. *That* is the important principle of **The poor, misunderstood calorie** alluded to above.

The Larson-Meyer energy deficit study didn't make it into the nutrient partitioning chapter because there were only very slight hints of a nutrient partitioning effect. But that is precisely what would be expected from the type of exercise intervention they performed. In other words, light aerobic exercise (group 3) is *modestly* better for body composition than diet alone. Groups 2 and 4 were treated with diet alone. Groups 2 and 3 lost approximately 10% of their body weight while group 4 lost approximately 14%, which was the predetermined amount of weight loss prescribed to group 4. Accordingly, group 4 lost the most fat mass (31% compared to 23% and 24% in groups 2 and 3, respectively). However, the amount of muscle lost by the exercising group (group 3) was modestly less than any other group. The absolute changes were small, but on a relative basis, group 3 (12.5% exercise + 12.5% diet) lost 20-33% less muscle mass than groups 1 (25% calorie restriction) and 3 (15% weight loss via diet alone). The small absolute differences were expected because aerobic exercise is not as good as anaerobic resistance exercise in nutrient partitioning or preserving lean mass.

Creating a 25% energy deficit by diet alone caused the subjects in group 2 to lose 8.4 kg. 69% of that was from fat mass. On the ultra-low calorie diet, subjects in group 4 lost 11 kg. 74% of that was from fat mass. When half of the 25% energy deficit was created by exercising, subjects in group 3 lost 8.1 kg and 78% of it came from fat mass. Thus, the small amount of exercise performed in group 3 was enough to enhance fat loss to a greater degree than that seen with a similar total energy deficit produced by diet alone. In other words, group 3's prescribed energy deficit was the same as group 2's, and they both lost the same amount of weight; so they were definitely both experiencing a similar energy deficit, but group 3 lost proportionately more fat. Subjects in group 3 **lost more fat mass without a more negative energy balance** *because of exercise*.

calories proper

11 β-hydroxysteroid dehydrogenase (11βHSD)

Dysregulation of glucocorticoid metabolism can have profound effects on energy balance. Cortisone is secreted from the adrenal glands during stress and is converted into the active metabolite cortisol by 11βHSD**1** within peripheral tissues. Via ligation of the glucocorticoid receptor, the tissue-specific effects of cortisol are:

I.   Hyperglycemia
   a. Adipose tissue: lipolysis
   b. Skeletal muscle:
      i. Proteolysis
      ii. Reduced glucose uptake
   c. Liver: gluconeogenesis

II. Anti-inflammatory
   a. Immune system suppression

III. Mineralocorticoid-like
   a. Mimics aldosterone
   b. Hypertension, hypokalemia

With regard to point III above, cortisol can bind to the mineralocorticoid or aldosterone receptor and cause fluid retention. However, mineralocorticoid-target tissues such as the kidney possess another enzyme, 11βHSD**2**, which *de*activates cortisol. 11βHSD**1** activates cortisol in liver, while 11βHSD**2** deactivates cortisol in the kidney. Because of these two enzymes, the levels of cortisol in the blood are not very meaningful; what matters is the amount of active cortisol within tissues, not necessarily the amount circulating in the blood.

Since cortisol has been associated with visceral fat accumulation, insulin resistance, and many comorbidities of obesity, one group engineered a line of mice to have more 11βHSD**1** selectively in adipose tissue (Masuzaki, Paterson et al. 2001). These mice were identical to normal mice with the exception of altered cortisol metabolism in fat tissue. To make a long story short, these mice weighed ~13% more, ate ~13% more, and had 64% more fat mass. Furthermore, they had over two times more visceral fat. Remember the only thing different about these mice was hormone signaling specifically in the fat cells. Altering the metabolism of adipose tissue by genetically increasing its capacity to accumulate fat *caused* an increase in food intake. The fat cell wanted to grow, so it sent a signal to the brain to eat more food so that it *could* grow. The cause and effect appear to be reversed, but it is the only logical explanation since the defect started in fat tissue. In these mice, to say 'increased food intake caused an increase in fat mass' is missing a critical point. **That is, the fat mass *caused* an increase in food intake.** Adipose tissue that is more susceptible to accumulate fat mass can cause an increase in appetite so that it *can* accumulate more fat mass; indeed, this is precisely what insulin does to adipose tissue.

Moving on, the reverse experiment was also performed whereby a line of mice was engineered to lack 11βHSD**1** (Morton, Paterson et al. 2004). Surprisingly, 11βHSD**1** knockout mice actually ate more food than wild-type, just like the 11βHSD**1** overexpressing mice. This might be an example of the importance of proper 'cortisol balance;' too much *or* too little cortisol activity can dysregulate appetite. However, these mice actually weighed less because of an intrinsically higher core body temperature (increased energy expenditure). They also stored more fat in subcutaneous depots and less in the viscera than their wild-type counterparts. As expected, given their reduced fat mass, 11βHSD**1** knockout mice had lower leptin levels which explains why they ate more, but not why they had increased energy expenditure (lower leptin levels would be predicted to reduce energy expenditure). To that end, the researchers concluded that altered fat distribution, with less visceral fat and more subcutaneous was the most likely cause for the improved metabolic profile in 11βHSD**1** knockout mice. Collectively, these studies suggest a critical role for hormones, independent of food intake, in the relationship between fat mass, appetite, and energy balance.

Trans fats; they also work in monkeys

There is no uniform protocol for monitoring energy balance in a research setting. In a diet study on African green monkeys (Kavanagh, Jones et al. 2007), researchers attempted to maintain energy balance by providing exactly 70 kcal per kg of body weight. They then measured body weight and adiposity for the next 6 years. Importantly, the monkeys were weighed at the beginning of the study, and this initial body weight measurement was used to determine their calorie intake for the following 6 years (just like Li's 5% calorie restricted mice above; food allocations were determined from baseline values). At the beginning of the study, the monkeys weighed ~6.5 kg (14.3 pounds);

for the rest of the study they were fed precisely
455 kilocalories every day. The diet was as follows:

	fat	protein	carbs	kcal
%	35%	17%	48%	455
g	18	9	24	

The diet for half of the monkeys was
supplemented with 8%, or ~4 grams of trans-fats.
The average intake for humans is 3% which is
approximately 7 grams per day. 8% per day for
humans would be approximately 18 grams, which
is on the high end but could easily be accomplished
by eating fast food or microwave popcorn a few
times per week. So besides being informative and
shedding an intriguing new light on energy balance,
this study is also of practical relevance. The
composition of the trans fat added was similar to
what is found in fast food: partially hydrogenated
soybean oil.

After 6 years, body weight in the control
group hadn't changed much. They weighed 6.41 kg
at baseline and 6.55 kg at follow-up, a change of
~2%. This was expected because at baseline, 70
kcal/d was enough food to keep them weight
stable, so essentially nothing changed in these
monkeys. More specifically, since food intake *and*

body weight didn't change, we can say that there were probably no major perturbations in energy balance in this group.

The trans fat group, on the other hand, gained almost 3 times more weight despite eating exactly the same amount of food as the control group, which was exactly the same amount of food they were eating when they were weight stable at baseline. Energy balance was clearly perturbed by trans fats. This excess weight was primarily in the form of increased visceral fat. In all, they had 27% more fat tissue than the control group. Fasting glucose and insulin levels were unchanged but postprandial insulin levels were markedly elevated in trans fat-fed monkeys compared to controls, suggesting that dietary trans fats indeed *caused* insulin resistance. **They gained a significant amount of fat mass despite an absence of excess calories.** This was most likely caused by the trans fat-induced insulin resistance and subsequent postprandial hyperinsulinemia.

They gained a significant amount of fat mass despite an absence of excess calories.

To recap,

-bedridden patients expend less energy but their appetite declines so they eat less and remain weight stable (or even lose weight). However these patients oftentimes end up with a higher body fat percentage because of the loss of lean mass. **They get fatter without a positive energy balance.**

-Li's 5% caloric restricted mice: whether they were fed 5% less than baseline or 5% less than control, they got fatter. **The mice got fatter despite eating less.**

-Type I diabetics are usually lean but develop fat deposits around their insulin injection sites. **Fat mass grew because of the hormonal milieu, not energy balance per se.**

-Subjects in Larson-Meyer's 12.5% diet + 12.5% exercise group lost more fat mass relative to muscle mass despite a similar energy deficit as the other groups. **They lost more fat mass without a more negative energy balance** *because of exercise.*

-11bHSD1 fat-specific overexpressing mice possess adipose tissue that is genetically driven to accumulate fat. **Growth of the fat tissue caused food intake to increase.**

-Kavanaugh's trans fat-fed monkeys **gained significantly more fat mass despite an absence of excess calories.**

What is the general theme underlying all of these findings? A calorie is not a calorie because energy balance doesn't matter. You can get fatter without eating more; you can even get fatter by eating less.

Obesity no longer requires a positive energy balance.

A new philosophy on energy balance

If someone were to match their 2,000 kilocalorie energy expenditure with 1,900 kilocalories of food intake and 100 kilocalories from adipose-derived fat calories, would we say they were in energy balance? In this example, *energy in* refers to the energy from food ingested today and the energy from excess food ingested in the past. This person would be losing fat mass despite being in apparent energy balance.

Is this why low carb diets tend to be hypocaloric? Low insulin levels would enhance lipolysis and lead to a net efflux of stored energy from adipose in the form of fatty acids. In other words, the brain probably doesn't know that 1,900 kilocalories came from the diet and 100 kilocalories came from adipose-derived fat… therefore the brain might only be hungry for 1,900 dietary kilocalories even though energy expenditure is 2,000 kilocalories.

Alternatively, what if someone ingests 2,000 kilocalories *and* releases 100 kilocalories from adipose-derived fat… and maybe they expend an additional 100 kilocalories that day by fidgeting, heat, or futile cycles. They would lose fat mass, but were they in energy balance? They were hungry for 2,000 kilocalories but the added energy released from adipose boosted energy expenditure. In other words, what if access to those calories from adipose *caused* the increase in energy expenditure; if those 100 kilocalories weren't released from adipose, then that person wouldn't have expended an additional 100 kilocalories that day.

When are they in energy balance?

Hunger for 2,000 kilocalories when energy expenditure is 2,000 kilocalories is considered appropriate. But what if the diet is low carb, so insulin stays low and more energy is released from adipose causing increased energy expenditure. Does this mean appetite was actually suppressed in this person?

Food for thought.

Chapter 13.
Carbs make fat people fatter

If all calories were created equal, then the biological response to a caloric load would be independent from its macronutrient composition. Furthermore, the response of two different people to the same caloric load would also be similar. But this is not the case.

The following examples come from overfeeding studies. The obesity epidemic was not caused by the sort of overfeeding used in these studies; it was much more likely caused by small fluctuations in nutrient partitioning compounded over time. Overfeeding studies try to condense the journey from lean to obese into a couple weeks. It is not physiological... But that doesn't mean overfeeding studies are irrelevant. On the contrary, some of these studies provide great insight into the complex interactions between diet, energy balance, and nutrient partitioning.

One study was done to compare the effects of two weeks of overfeeding either fat or carbohydrates in lean and obese subjects (Horton, Drougas et al. 1995). In this study, the baseline diet was kept the same in all treatments, but total calories were increased 50% with either all carbohydrates or all fat. The caloric requirements for weight maintenance in lean and obese subjects were ~2,700 and ~3,300 kcal/d, respectively.

During overfeeding, lean and obese subjects consumed 4,000 and 5,000 kcal/d, respectively.

Kcal/d

	lean	obese
maintenance	2,657	3,336
overfeeding	3,986	5,004

The overfeeding period lasted 2 weeks and this study was designed as a crossover. This means that each subject receives both treatments separated by a washout period (~4 weeks). This is the best kind of study design because it essentially allows each subject to be compared to themself; it controls for almost every conceivable potentially confounding factors.

Energy expenditure was assessed by whole-room indirect calorimetry in order to determine how much excess energy was expended, how much was stored, as well as the form of stored energy (fat or glycogen). The obese subjects had a chronically higher level of food intake, but their energy expenditure was normal per unit of lean body mass; thus, they were weight stable but at a higher body weight than the lean subjects.

Baseline characteristics

	lean	obese
BW (kg)	68	104
fat (kg)	15	37
body fat (%)	21%	36%
FFM (kg)	54	67
kcal/kg FFM	49	50

After 3 weeks of 50% overfeeding, body weight increased by about 3 kg (6.6 pounds) in both groups, with slightly greater increases during carbohydrate compared to fat overfeeding. And most of the excess was stored as fat mass in both groups regardless of what was being overfed. The researchers estimated that ~75% of the excess energy was stored.

Here are some rough estimates of the diet during each phase of the experiment:

Maintenance diet

	lean	obese
kcal/d	2,657	3,336
fat %	36%	33%
fat (g)	106	122
CHO (%)	49%	52%
CHO (g)	326	434

Obese subjects ingested more calories than lean subjects, but the macronutrient composition was similar.

Carbohydrate overfeeding was accomplished by eating 283 additional grams of carbs in the lean group for a total of 609 grams per day, and 355 additional grams of carbs per day in the obese group for a total of 789 grams of carbs per day:

carbohydrate overfeeding

	lean	obese
kcal/d	3,986	5,004
fat %	24%	22%
fat (g)	106	122
CHO (%)	61%	63%
CHO (g)	609	789

_____

_____

_____

_____

_____

_____

_____

_____

Fat overfeeding was accomplished by eating 148 additional grams of fat in the lean group, for a total of 254 grams per day, and 185 additional grams of fat per day in the obese group, for a total of 308 grams of fat per day:

fat overfeeding

	lean	obese
kcal/d	3,986	5,004
fat %	57%	55%
fat (g)	254	308
CHO (%)	33%	35%
CHO (g)	326	434

Importantly, neither diet was deficient in any macronutrient; although all of the excess calories during the fat overfeeding phase were from fat, the diet still contained 326-434 grams of carbohydrates (same as the maintenance diet). The proportion of calories derived from carbohydrates decreased from ~50% to ~34% but this was not a low carb diet. In other words, there was still enough carbs in both diets to stimulate insulin secretion in both groups to divert a majority of the excess energy ingested into adipose tissue.

The amount of fat stored during the fat overfeeding phase was primarily determined by the energy balance. Both lean and obese people gained a similar amount of fat relative to what they were consuming during this phase. However, interestingly, the same was not true for carbohydrate overfeeding. The amount of fat stored during carbohydrate overfeeding increased with body weight. Obese subjects stored more of the excess energy as fat during carbohydrate overfeeding than lean people. Excess carbs were more fattening to obese subjects compared to their lean counterparts. **Thus, carbs made fat people fatter.** Part of this may be due to the fact that obese subjects tended to have a higher respiratory quotient than lean subjects, meaning that they oxidized relatively more glucose than fat compared to a lean subject; in other words, the obese metabolism preferentially oxidizes glucose regardless of how much fat is in the diet. When the obese subjects ate more glucose, yes, glucose oxidation increased, but at the expense of fat oxidation. Therefore, to provoke an obese metabolism to burn more fat, a greater carbohydrate restriction is required than would be necessary for a lean metabolism. Carbs were less fattening for lean subjects; they maintained a lower respiratory quotient, reflecting more fat oxidation compared to obese subjects.

The fat mass data were confirmed, albeit on a much shorter timescale (3 days), by McDevitt and colleagues (McDevitt, Poppitt et al. 2000) who showed that carbohydrate overfeeding caused a greater positive fat balance in obese compared to lean subjects.

The carbohydrate oxidation data were confirmed by an overfeeding study similar to Horton's(Diaz, Prentice et al. 1992). In this study, lean and overweight subjects were overfed by half for 6 weeks and underwent a battery of physical and biochemical tests. The diet was 12% protein, 42% fat, and 46% carbohydrates. During the overfeeding period, both groups gained roughly

10% of their bodyweight comprised of 1/3 muscle and 2/3 fat. Fat oxidation is suppressed by carbohydrate ingestion. Fat oxidation was suppressed by 37% in lean subjects during the overfeeding period and by almost twice that in obese subjects (~64%). Carbohydrates were more fattening in obese subjects compared to lean subjects in Horton's study. In Diaz's study, carbohydrate overfeeding suppressed fat oxidation to a much greater extent in obese subjects compared to lean subjects. This shouldn't be interpreted to mean that obese patients have an intrinsic disadvantage or weak spot when it comes to the fattening effect of dietary carbohydrates, it should be interpreted to mean that they have an advantage when it comes to fat loss; carbohydrate restriction will provide relatively greater benefits to an obese patient relative to a lean one.

The "carbs are more fattening for obese subjects" findings of Horton and "carbs suppress fat oxidation to a greater extent in obese subjects" findings of Diaz are further confirmed by a non-overfeeding study where obese and lean women were fed either a low carb or low fat eucaloric (weight-maintaining) diet for 4 weeks (Roust, Hammel et al. 1994). On the low-carb diet, obese women exhibited a lower respiratory quotient than lean women, meaning that they were burning relatively more fat. On the low-fat diet, obese women exhibited a higher respiratory quotient than lean women, meaning that they were burning relative less fat. If fuel selection was simply a matter of availability, then respiratory quotient would be the same in lean and obese women. But it's not. These findings suggest that on a low fat high carb diet, obese subjects will be:

1. burning less fat than lean subjects according to Roust's & Diaz's study

2. gaining more fat than lean subjects according to Horton's & McDevitt's studies

These studies demonstrate an aspect of energy balance that is key to nutrient partitioning. Given the same amount of excess dietary energy intake, obese people will accumulate more fat mass than lean people if that excess energy is carbohydrates. Obese people stand to benefit more from carbohydrate restriction than lean people in terms of fat loss.

Why does this happen? It's not entirely clear, but there are some hints. Tremblay and colleagues performed a series of great overfeeding studies. In one analysis (Tremblay, Nadeau et al. 1995), they divided the subjects into two groups based on their insulin responsivity: 'high responders' secreted more insulin in response to overfeeding than 'low responders.' They found that high responders gained significantly more fat mass during overfeeding than low responders. This was confirmed in another study which showed that insulin response to a glucose load (at baseline) was positively correlated to the increase in fat mass during a 3 month overfeeding period (Oppert, Nadeau et al. 1995). Furthermore, these findings are in agreement with the known anabolic effects of insulin on fat tissue.

If insulin responsivity is indeed to blame, what determines one's insulin responsivity? More insulin is secreted in response to a meal in insulin resistant subjects, but they are usually overweight, so which comes first? Tremblay's findings imply insulin resistance precedes the development of obesity, whereas Horton's findings imply obesity precedes carbohydrate intolerance. In Horton's overfeeding study, more fat mass at baseline correlated with greater fat deposition in response to high carbohydrate overfeeding.

Which comes first, obesity or insulin resistance, is of minor fundamental importance because the cure is well-established (carbohydrate restriction). However, there is still much debate and research into more proximal solutions; perhaps carbohydrates, per se, are not the sole cause of insulin resistance and obesity. It is possible that specific carbohydrates or carb-rich foods are to blame. Maybe carbohydrate restriction should apply preferentially to fructose or grains. These issues have not been entirely resolved as of the writing of this book, and I expect it will be quite a while before they are.

Carbs still make lean people fat

In the meantime, carbs might also make lean people fat. Remember the Women's Health Initiative? (one of the biggest diet studies ever conducted, ~40,000 women, over 7 years of follow-up). In brief, the intervention was designed to reduce fat intake, and it did, by almost 25%. Total calorie intake declined slightly while physical activity increased slightly. However, the carbohydrates increased from 45% to 53%. The difference is admittedly very small, but may have been relevant: a follow-up study provided interesting insight into one of the original subgroup analyses (Tinker, Bonds et al. 2008). In the original study, the low fat *higher carb* diet actually caused the subgroup of women who were lean at baseline to gain weight. On average, total caloric intake declined and physical activity increased; the researchers didn't measure *total* energy expenditure, but it probably declined. Did these women gain weight be*cause* of a relatively minor increase in dietary carbohydrates sustained for the entire study duration? Obesity doesn't happen overnight, and these women were overweight, not obese. Yet.

Furthermore, lean people like those mentioned above have a lower BMI (by definition), higher insulin sensitivity, and a lower risk for diabetes than overweight or obese people. In a follow-up analysis of the original data, Tinker and colleagues showed that women with a lower BMI and higher insulin sensitivity at baseline actually had a slightly greater risk of developing diabetes if they were assigned to the low fat *higher carb* group.

Chapter 14.
Nutrient Partitioning

Nutrient partitioning is probably the single most important factor supporting the most positive possible outcome in a long-term weight loss strategy (and it is one of my favorite concepts in nutritional biochemistry and physiology). "Build muscle and burn fat." Essentially, nutrient partitioning is the antithesis of "getting fat without a positive energy balance."

Generally, the principles of energy balance and nutrient partitioning are universal. Therefore, to make the broadest case possible, I have included a wide variety of examples including men and women, lean and obese, diseased and healthy, and animal models.

Insulin

Managing insulin is a key component of nutrient partitioning. Insulin promotes fuel storage; i.e., it causes fat storage in adipose tissue and glucose storage as glycogen in skeletal muscle. In adipose tissue, insulin enhances fat uptake by stimulating the enzyme *lipoprotein lipase*. It also prevents the release of fatty acids ("lipolysis") by inhibiting the enzyme *hormone-sensitive lipase*. Hormone-sensitive lipase is aptly named; it is extremely sensitive to the effects of insulin (it is said to be the most "hormone-sensitive" enzyme in the body). In other words, it only takes a little bit of insulin to completely inhibit lipolysis. On the other hand, insulin has anabolic (muscle-building) effects on skeletal muscle. Thus, we want to minimize the effect of insulin on fat storage in adipose while maximizing it on anabolism in muscle. To put things into perspective, however, the effects of insulin on fat storage are quantitatively more robust than its effects on muscle anabolism.

Leucine

Keeping insulin levels low, by following a low glycemic index diet or simply reducing carbohydrate intake facilitates fat burning. The caveat: low insulin means less anabolic effects on muscle. Fortunately, there is an easy way around this. Enter: Leucine. The essential amino acid leucine has an anabolic effect on muscle comparable to insulin. Leucine is present at high levels in whey protein, and is thought to be one of the primary contributors to the anabolic effect of whey protein. Leucine and increased dietary protein can compensate for the effects of low insulin on skeletal muscle. And even though some proteins are modestly insulinogenic, dietary protein does not promote net fat storage.

The biological rationale for leucine supplementation is strong. One of the major leucine studies was done in healthy elderly adult men (Verhoeven, Vanschoonbeek et al. 2009). In this study, they recruited a group of healthy men and had them consume 2.5 grams of leucine with every meal for 3 months. 3 months is a relatively short time period and 7.5 grams is a moderate dose. At baseline and follow-up the researchers performed a battery of strength and body composition tests. To make a long story short, leucine supplementation did not perform well in this study. While trying to explain why no effect was seen, some of the critics of this study pointed out that the protein synthetic response to leucine is blunted in elderly patients, so the results might be different in a younger population or with a higher dose.

Alternatively, these were consuming roughly 2,000 kilocalories daily with 17%, or ~83 grams of protein. This amounts to ~1 g/kg, which is above the minimum requirements of 0.8 g/kg. In other words, they had a high baseline protein and thus leucine intake; therefore an additional 7.5 grams was relatively not very much.

Interestingly, the authors performed a comprehensive plasma amino acid analysis every two weeks for the entire study and found very few dramatic changes. Plasma leucine went from 105 μM to 115 μM in both leucine *and* placebo groups. Again, this may be due to the fact that these men had a high baseline protein intake, but those findings stand in contrast to the results from Crowe and colleagues, who conducted a very similar study (Crowe, Weatherson et al. 2006). Crowe recruited a cohort of young healthy athletes and administered about half the dose used by Verhoeven, ~3.3 grams per day for 6 weeks. Besides finding robust improvements in a variety of measures of athletic performance (total work output, peak power production, time to exhaustion, etc.), they observed a significant increase in plasma leucine from 140 μM to 160 μM. The athletes in Crowe's study were consuming surprisingly much less protein than Verhoeven's elderly men, 0.85 g/kg compared to 1 g/kg. Neither group found any effect on body composition, but leucine supplementation in young athletes with a low habitual protein intake significantly enhanced athletic performance. With increased work output, power production, and time to exhaustion, the subjects in Crowe's study would most definitely see improvements in body composition after a few months.

Exogenous hormones

Growth hormone

Growth hormone is secreted from the anterior pituitary of the brain and provides an anabolic signal to many tissues of the body. In combination with thyroid hormone, growth hormone triggers anabolic effects in muscle. To provide the energy for skeletal muscle hypertrophy, growth hormone stimulates lipolysis in adipose tissue. Thus, growth hormone builds muscle and burns fat (the archetypal "nutrient partitioner"). Growth hormone is also a counter-regulatory hormone, meaning it prevents hypoglycemia. In this regard, it is considered 'anti-insulin.' Growth hormone has been abused by athletes but it is more commonly used in the farming and agriculture industries for its nutrient partitioning effects. I do not advocate the use of growth hormone to achieve nutrient partitioning, but I think it is a great example of how the hormonal milieu can manipulate the building and burning of muscle and adipose, respectively, independent from changes in energy balance.

For example, in one long-term study, a cohort of 49 male and female patients were prescribed 0.5 - 1.0 mg of growth hormone (6-12 μg/kg;) daily and followed for 42 months (Jorgensen, Fougner et al. 2011). Growth hormone's primary effect is to increase IGF-1 levels and the patients receiving growth hormone experienced an increase in IGF-1 from 10 nM to 25 nM, which simply confirmed that the growth hormone treatment worked. Although the main outcome was quality of life measurements, which improved drastically, there were considerable improvements in body composition. Keep in mind that there was *no dietary intervention*. The patients began and finished the study weighing approximately 83 kg, meaning that they were weight-stable and thus in energy balance over the course of three and a half years. The important findings were that their initial body fat levels of ~32% were reduced to 28%. Thus, their fat mass declined by >10% due to the hormone treatment. Conversely, muscle mass increased by 3%. In other words, **they gained muscle and lost fat without a**

change in energy balance. This is, by definition, nutrient partitioning. These findings also confirm (or merely *suggest* [to be proper]) that quality of life is correlated with muscle mass. Furthermore, this demonstrates that a particular hormonal milieu, in this example elevated growth hormone, is capable of regulating fat mass *independent of energy balance*. This is one of the main principles of **The poor, misunderstood calorie**.

A study into the effects of growth hormone was done in patients with low baseline growth hormone levels and even though the study was of shorter duration, the results were more dramatic (Salomon, Cuneo et al. 1989). In this study, 24 subjects were recruited and divided evenly into a placebo or active treatment group. The treatment group self-administered a dose of 0.07 U/kg (27 µg/kg; ~2.2 mg) of growth hormone subcutaneously every night for 6 months. Baseline IGF-1 levels were 0.41 nM, much lower than in Jorgensen's population confirming that these subjects had chronically low growth hormone. Treatment increased their IGF-1 levels over three-fold to 1.53 nM.

The researchers used total body potassium to determine lean body mass. Lean body mass contains approximately 3 grams or 66 millimoles of potassium per kilogram and it is almost entirely stored in lean tissue. A portion, 0.0118%, of this potassium is in the form of a naturally occurring isotope potassium-40, which can be detected by a device known as a gamma counter. It is a very expensive but very accurate technique.

The subjects weighed 81 kg (~178 pounds) at baseline with 50 kg (~110 pounds) of lean body mass and ~38% body fat. Basal metabolic rate was assessed by indirect calorimetry and was ~1,664 kcal/d. After 6 months of treatment, body weight did not change in either group. Body fat, on the other hand, decreased dramatically by 16% *despite no change in body weight*. They gained 6.2 kg (almost 14 pounds) of lean body mass. As expected, given that lean body mass is the main driver of energy expenditure, basal metabolic rate increased by 16% to 1,931 kcal/d. This increase was greater than expected; their normalized metabolic rate at baseline was 32.4 kcal/kg of lean body mass. After treatment it increased to 34.4. If the increase in absolute metabolic rate was due solely to the increased lean body mass, then this ratio would not have changed. The increase in relative metabolic rate (kcal/kg lean body mass) means they had more muscle mass and this increased muscle mass was more metabolically active. This probably contributed to the astounding reduction in body fat experienced by these subjects. Growth hormone stimulates lipolysis in adipose tissue and hypertrophy in skeletal muscle. Thus, it increases the amount of free fatty acids in the blood and enhances the capacity for them to be burned by creating more muscle tissue. All of this can occur during a state of energy balance, and this is the essence of nutrient partitioning. Their metabolic rate increased, but they remained weight stable; they were actually eating more food but the new[19] hormonal milieu facilitated muscle growth and fat oxidation. Furthermore, given that part of growth hormone's physiological effects come from its insulin antagonism, these effects can be partially recapitulated by reducing insulin levels via carbohydrate restriction to enhance lipolysis, and increasing protein intake and performing resistance exercise to enhance muscle growth.

Cjc-1295

Growth hormone secretion is pulsatile. That is, its concentration ranges from 5 ng/mL during the daytime all the way up to 45 ng/mL about an hour after falling asleep. It is regulated by

---

[19] Dare I say "more optimal"

a wide variety of factors. Normal growth hormone therapy, like that used by Jorgensen, consists of injecting growth hormone directly so that the levels are elevated around the clock. A compound known as cjc-1295 is a growth hormone secretagogue, and it potentiates the pulsatile peaks of growth hormone. In other words, it is more like natural growth hormone but with an umph.

A recent study examined cjc-1295 in AIDs patients. (Falutz, Allas et al. 2005). AIDS patients tend to have poor musculature and lipodystrophy (abnormal adipose tissue deposition). Over the course of 12 weeks, 61 patients self-administered subcutaneous injections of placebo or 2 mg cjc-1295 daily. In accord with Jorgensen's findings, IGF-1 was increased in all treatment groups confirming the GH mimetic effects of cjc-1295. IFG-1 increased from 2.9 nM in placebo to 10.3 nM and 13.4 nM in the 1 mg and 2 mg groups, respectively. Although the absolute levels of IGF-1 were lower in these patients compared to those in Jorgensen's study, the magnitude of increase was larger (4.6 vs. 2.5-fold), confirming the potency of cjc-1295. There was no dietary intervention or food intake measurements, and body weight was similar and unaffected by treatment in all 3 groups. Fat mass, on the other hand, increased 1.4% in the placebo group and was reduced by 8% due to cjc-1295. Furthermore, muscle mass declined by 0.5 kg in the placebo group but increased 1.7 kg in the treatment groups. Although no attempt was made to quantify any aspect of energy balance, we know that body weight was stable, fat mass declined, and muscle mass increased in the treatment group. Cjc-1295 does not have a magical, non-physiological mechanism of action; it merely tweaks growth hormone secretion. In other words, **minor shifts in hormone levels have the ability to completely remodel the metabolic landscape and induce profound changes in body composition** *independent of energy balance*. Furthermore, it is frankly wrong to attribute 'getting fat' to a simple caloric surplus.

Ephedrine

Ephedrine was once considered the holy grail of all weight loss supplements for its unmatched effects on nutrient partitioning and body composition. Ephedrine acts on beta-adrenergic receptors in fat tissue to stimulate lipolysis. This increases the release of free fatty acids, which is only beneficial if those free fatty acids are utilized. Ephedrine also stimulated the sympathetic nervous system, elevating energy expenditure and increasing fatty acid oxidation. Moreover, ephedrine exhibited a remarkable "muscle-sparing" effect that is very desirable for individuals trying to lose weight.

Although it has been around for thousands of years, ephedrine has received a lot of bad press lately. However, I would like to discuss ephedrine as another example of how nutrient partitioning can alter body composition independently from energy balance, not to advocate its use.

Ephedrine's muscle sparing properties are best exemplified in the arena of weight loss. One early study (Buemann, Marckmann et al. 1994) looked into the use of ephedrine in a population of overweight but otherwise healthy women. The dose was 20mg three times per day, and they were followed for 12 weeks. Food intake was not measured, but the subjects were instructed to 'go about their usual routine.' While this complicates interpreting the data in the context of nutrient partitioning, the results were quite robust. At study entry, the women weighed ~66.3 kg (146 lbs) and had ~33% body fat. By 12 weeks they lost almost 10% (12 pounds!) of their initial body weight. Just for some perspective, that is a huge amount of weight to lose in such a short amount of time. Body fat was drastically reduced by 16% and fat free mass was virtually unscathed. On a percent basis, fat free mass actually increased from 66.9% to 72.1% of body weight. 91% of the weight lost was fat mass (!!). During a standard low fat diet, usually around 66% of the weight lost is fat mass; thus, ephedrine improved the efficiency of fat loss by almost half.

This study suffers from lack of a proper control group and insufficient dietary information, but it quite clearly demonstrates that in a free-living population, ephedrine selectively and profoundly targets fat mass for destruction. In other words, **the regulation of fat mass is not restricted to deviations in energy balance**; this is a key principle of **The poor, misunderstood calorie**.

A similar study was done in a population of lean and obese male rhesus monkeys (Ramsey, Colman et al. 1998). This study lasted 8 weeks and used a dose of 18 mg ephedrine per day, or approximately 1.15 mg/kg, which is very similar on a weight basis to the dose used by Astrup (60 mg/day ≈ 0.9 mg/kg). These animals were also given 150 mg caffeine which is about the amount of caffeine in one small cup of coffee. After 8 weeks of treatment, obese monkeys that started the study weighing ~16 kg (34 lbs) with 25% body fat lost ~8% of their initial body weight and almost 20% of their initial fat mass. 82% of the weight lost was fat. That is not as much as the women in Astrup's study, in whom 91% of the weight lost was fat; this was most likely due to a species difference, but also could have been due to a gender difference or Ramsey's inclusion of caffeine for the rhesus monkeys. In any case, 82% is still better than the 66% achieved by low fat diets. Total energy expenditure increased ~10% from 905 kcal/d to 977 kcal/d during treatment *and* food intake was suppressed despite the marked decrease in leptin from 10 µg/L down to 5 µg/L. The reduction in leptin *should have* signaled to the brain that there was an energy deficit and it's time to eat more, but ephedrine is a powerful appetite suppressant.

This study also used a group of lean monkeys and the results shed a particularly interesting light on the regulation of energy balance. For starters, the lean monkeys weighing 10 kg (22 lbs) had only a fraction of the body fat of obese monkeys (7% vs. 25%). Energy expenditure increased significantly more in lean than obese monkeys (20% vs. 10%), although this was most likely due to the higher relative dose of ephedrine. 18 mg for an obese 16 kg monkey = 1.15 mg/kg; for a lean 10 kg monkey = 1.74 mg/kg. However, the increase in energy expenditure was *two times greater* in lean monkeys, while the dose was only half greater, suggesting obesity may confer resistance to sympathetic nervous system activation.

There were fundamental differences in the physiological responses to ephedrine in lean compared to obese monkeys. The lean monkeys lost 0.07 kg of body weight, significantly less than obese monkeys despite taking a higher relative dose. But this may have been expected because of their drastically lower initial fat mass; they still lost a similar relative amount of fat (21% vs. 19% in lean and obese, respectively). Interestingly, the lean monkeys ate more and actually gained muscle mass during the treatment. The lean monkeys ate more than they were eating prior to treatment which was also more than obese monkeys during treatment. Usually, increasing food intake increases both fat and muscle mass, however due to ephedrine's selective targeting of adipose tissue, ephedrine was burning the fat while the energy from the increased food intake was being invested into muscle tissue. Lean monkeys were also more physically active, which is known to facilitate nutrient partitioning (like exercise). Thus, these monkeys ate more food, gained lean muscle mass, and lost body fat. Sounds like a pretty good deal, right?

If body composition were strictly a matter of energy balance, it would be impossible to increase muscle and decrease fat simultaneously; you'd either be in a negative energy balance, which would burn fat and waste muscle, or a positive energy balance, which would increase fat mass and build muscle. Ephedrine tweaked the autonomic nervous system which facilitated nutrient partitioning. Overall they lost weight, so technically they were in a negative energy balance. **The monkeys gained muscle and burned fat despite being in negative energy balance**.

Nutrient timing

Elevated insulin levels occur more frequently on a low-fat than a low-carb diet due simply to the quantities of carbohydrates in the respective diets. Chronically elevated insulin leads to a much greater stimulation of fat storage than, for example, insulin elevated only in short bursts. Therefore, eating a diet consisting mainly of complete proteins, vegetables (of course), and high quality fats for most of the day, while consuming protein and moderate amounts of carbohydrates around the time of exercise might be an optimal example of 'nutrient partitioning' on a mixed diet.

The effect of nutrient timing of protein ingestion on muscle hypertrophy has been examined in a variety of paradigms. For example, in one study (Esmarck, Andersen et al. 2001), 13 men underwent a 12 week resistance training program with either drinking a protein shake immediately after or two hours after exercise. The men were healthy and lean, and the exercise regimen was pretty good. It only lasted ~30 minutes and consisted of a 5 minute warm-up followed by 3 compound exercises[20]. Importantly, the researchers made sure intensity was high and they frequently increased the amount of weight each subject was lifting. The protein shake contained 10 grams of protein, 7 grams of carbohydrates, and 3.3 grams of fat. After 12 weeks, both groups improved, but the group ingesting protein immediately after exercise made significantly greater increases in muscular strength and power. Accordingly, skeletal muscles from the upper leg (quadriceps and hamstring) experienced

---

[20] Compound exercise- an exercise that utilizes multiple muscle groups, for example: squats, deadlifts, good mornings, etc.

a greater degree of hypertrophy in the group ingesting protein immediately after exercise compared to the group who ingested protein 2 hours later, who experienced very little hypertrophy. The group who ingested protein 2 hours later lost one kg of body weight and this was entirely from fat. Although there was no change in body weight in the group ingesting protein immediately after exercise, they increased muscle mass by 1 kg and decreased fat mass by 1 kg. In other words, protein timing exerted a direct nutrient partitioning effect. These changes were larger than expected in this study because, despite its short duration, the subjects only had a few weeks to learn the exercises before the study commenced. In other words, some of the gains they made were due to the 'athlete's learning curve.' But not the differences in body composition; since both groups were undergoing the same learning curve, the differences in body composition can only be explained by nutrient timing. Consuming a protein shake very close to the time of exercise causes those calories to be used differently compared to if they were ingested 2 hours later. The protein shake, and thus the "calories," were the same in both groups, but the body treated those calories differently because of *when* they were consumed. This would not happen in a bomb calorimeter. The right nutrient composition or **nutrient timing can cause fat loss and muscle gain independent from changes in energy balance**.

The results of a similar study from 2006 were considerably more robust than Esmarck's immediately vs. 2 hours post protein shake findings. In this study (Cribb and Hayes 2006), 23 young healthy men who knew their way around the gym were recruited. Given their weightlifting experience, there would have been very little 'learning curve' effect, but the researchers still gave them *12-weeks* to adapt to the new regimen! That is an extremely long time; perhaps they didn't want to lose any time because the intervention only ran for 10 weeks. The exercise training was high-intensity *overload* training designed to increase strength and muscle hypertrophy. These guys were pushed very hard. The protein shake contained 0.4 grams of whey protein per kilogram of body weight, which worked out to be roughly 32 grams of protein. Both groups exercised in the late afternoon and ate all of their meals at similar times of the day. The pre/post group consumed 1 protein shake immediately prior to exercise and another immediately afterwards. The morning/evening group consumed 1 protein shake before breakfast and another before bed.

For starters, that is a lot of protein. In addition to what they were initially consuming, the whey protein shakes added an extra 64 grams of protein per day. Not surprisingly, the increased dietary protein had a satiating effect in both groups; by the end of the study their total calorie intake was slightly lower than at baseline.

The effects of exercise are generally much more robust in naïve subjects, or those who have never exercised before. These guys were healthy and pretty strong at the beginning of the study, so we expect their response to be less than the general population. On average, strength increased by over 10% in all the subjects. Since they were all experienced exercisers, and the only thing that changed was the introduction of protein shakes, it can be concluded that the 10% strength gains came solely from the added daily protein and not nutrient timing. However, strength gains induced by ingesting the protein shakes immediately before and after exercise were 20% greater than those in the morning/evening group. Given the close correlation between muscle strength and function, these results would translate to marked improvements in quality of life.

In other words, if someone is unable to exercise at a very high intensity, they may be able to partially compensate by consuming a protein shake immediately before and after exercising.

Both groups experienced increased muscle gains. However, the guys in the morning/evening group gained ~1.4 kilograms of muscle with little change in fat mass. Guys in the pre/post group gained twice the amount of muscle and actually lost fat mass. Calorie and nutrient intake was similar between the groups. The only difference was nutrient timing. Simply drinking the protein shake *at a different time of the day* caused the calories to be diverted away from fat tissue and toward building muscle mass. **It's possible to alter body composition *while in energy balance* by changing not only what you eat, but when you eat it**.

Dietary protein, in general

Dietary protein is necessary to optimize the anabolic effects of exercise on muscle tissue. Consuming protein around the time of exercise targets the amino acids toward muscle due to the exercise-induced shift in blood flow. This is where protein supplements come in handy. Compared to whole food protein sources (chicken, eggs, meat, etc.), protein supplements are very convenient. Prepare one in advance, and sip on it on your way to the gym. By the time you start exercising, the amino acids will be entering the bloodstream. Muscle contractions will recruit a greater blood flow and divert a lot of the amino acids directly toward the exercising muscles to effectively optimize the anabolic effects of exercise.

Exercise

The intensity and duration of exercise are important determinants of fuel utilization. Most of these factors are measured in terms of oxygen consumption. "VO_2" is the volume of oxygen you breathe. VO_{2max} is the most you can breathe during heavy exercise and is used as a rough gauge of intensity. An athlete might have a VO_{2max} of 3 litres per minute, for example. VO_2 increases in parallel with exercise intensity until the VO_{2max} has been reached.   A cyclist riding at 100 watts might have a VO_2 of 1.5 litres of oxygen per minute. At 200 watts they are at 3.0 litres of oxygen per minute. This doesn't mean the cyclist can't ride any faster, it means they can't breathe any faster (but in general they really can't ride *that* much

faster when they have reached their VO_{2max}).
Watts are a measure of power use, equal to 1 joule
per second or 0.000239 kilocalories per second.
Riding a bike at 200 watts for 30 minutes requires
86 kilocalories:

200 watts x .000239 kcal/s = 0.0478 kcal/s

0.0478 kcal/s x 60 s/min x 30 min = 86 kcal

Actually, your body will require considerably more
than 86 kilocalories for that ride due to its inherent
inefficiency. For reference, an athlete riding very
fast can get up to 300 watts.

Similar to VO_{2max}, lactate threshold is
another gauge of athletic performance. Lactate is
increased during anaerobic glycolysis, or the non-
oxidative metabolism of glucose. This occurs
during high intensity exercise. Lactate levels rise
when production exceeds clearance, this usually
occurs when someone is working between 55% and
85% VO_{2max} depending on their training status.

As discussed above, exercise itself can
function as a nutrient partitioning agent. During
exercise, glucose is taken up selectively by the
exercising muscles. Insulin, on the other hand,
stimulates glucose uptake into fat *and* muscle

(glucose uptake into fat tissue promotes fat storage). Furthermore, exercise shifts blood flow away from adipose and toward the contracting muscles.   Nutrients consumed around the time of exercise are selectively taken up by muscle, due to this shift in blood flow. This also goes for fatty acids released from adipose tissue. Exercise stimulates the sympathetic nervous system which causes lipolysis in adipose tissue. Therefore, if you are going to consume carbs, doing so around the time of exercise will minimize their impact on fat storage in adipose by two mechanisms: contraction-induced muscle glucose uptake decreases the glucose available to 1) stimulate insulin secretion and 2) enter into adipose tissue and facilitate fat storage.

One study was done which inadvertently demonstrated this point (Ballor, McCarthy et al. 1990). 27 obese women were put on a 1,200 kilocalorie diet and assigned to one of two exercise programs. Both programs were designed to expend equal calories, but the first program was high intensity (85% VO_{2max}) for a short duration (25 minutes) and the second program was low intensity (45% VO_{2max}) for long duration (50 minutes). Each group trained 3 days per week for 8 weeks.

Recall that exercise at a higher % of VO_{2max}, or higher intensity, requires more glucose oxidation relative to fat oxidation. Since the two groups expended the same amount of calories during exercise, it would be predicted that the low intensity group would burn more fat overall compared to the high intensity group. Exercise at 45% VO_{2max} burns roughly equal amounts of fat and glucose. Exercise at 85% VO_{2max}, on the other hand, gets over 90% of its fuel requirements from glucose oxidation. At low intensity, the glucose that is oxidized is primarily from blood glucose. At high intensity, most of the glucose is from muscle glycogen. One last point is that as exercise duration increases there is a gradual shift to increased fat oxidation due to glycogen depletion and the hormonal stimulation of lipolysis.

Back to the study: The absolute level of intensity in the two groups, as per VO_2 (L/min) during exercise, was 2.11 for high intensity and 1.18 for low intensity. Peak heart rate was 165 beats per minute for high intensity and 127.5 for low intensity. Respiratory quotient was 0.92 for high intensity and 0.80 for low intensity. All of these things confirm that the exercises really did differ significantly in intensity. Higher intensity exercise requires greater oxygen consumption, faster heart rate, and burns more glucose compared to lower intensity exercise. But the critical factor in this study was energy expenditure. Both groups burned 270 kilocalories per session; the high intensity group just burned it at a much faster rate (10.4 vs. 5.7 kilocalories per minute)

It is important not to confuse high intensity *aerobic* exercise, e.g., running, with high intensity *anaerobic* exercise. High intensity aerobic exercise enhances endurance and improves cardiovascular function but takes a toll on skeletal muscle. High intensity anaerobic (resistance) exercise, on the other hand, promotes skeletal muscle hypertrophy. Both groups in this study were performing aerobic/endurance exercise, which is not optimal for maintaining or building muscle mass. However, the differences in exercise intensity did have a predictable effect on body composition.

After 8 weeks, the women in both groups lost approximately 6 kg, or 8% of their initial starting weight. VO_{2max} improved in both groups, confirming good adherence to the exercise regimen, and it improved significantly more in the high intensity group, confirming that they were working *harder*, albeit for a shorter duration. As expected, because we know that high intensity aerobic exercise causes skeletal muscle breakdown, the high intensity group lost more muscle than the low intensity group, despite expending a similar amount of energy on exercise. The low intensity group lost more fat mass (and less muscle) than the high intensity group. 75% of the weight lost came from fat in the high intensity group, while 84% of the weight lost came from fat in the low intensity group. Low intensity aerobic exercise selectively burned more fat and preserved lean mass compared to high intensity aerobic exercise.

From the respiratory quotient data, the authors were able to calculate the amount of glucose and fat oxidation during the two programs. They determined 74.1% of the energy expended, or 200 kilocalories, was derived from glucose oxidation in the high intensity group. Therefore, it can be extrapolated that exercising at 85% VO2max burns approximately 1.93 grams of glucose per minute. We are unable to estimate the contribution of protein oxidation, but if the difference was theoretically 100% fat, that would mean fat was burning at a rate of 299.7 mg per minute. In the low intensity group, 33.4% of the energy expended was glucose oxidation (471.7 mg/min) and if the rest were all fat, it would be 419.9 mg/min. Thus, the absolute rate of fat oxidation is over 33% greater for low intensity aerobic exercise compared to high intensity aerobic exercise. The low intensity group oxidized approximately 21 grams of fat per session, multiplied by 3 sessions per week and 8 weeks equals 504 grams of fat (4,535 kcal). The high intensity group burned 180 grams of fat (1,619 kcal). Therefore, the low intensity group burned 2,916 kcal of fat (324 grams) more than the high intensity group. Take home message: low intensity, long duration, aerobic exercise (45% VO_{2max}, heart rate 127.5 bpm, duration 50 minutes) is more effective for nutrient partitioning than high intensity, short duration, aerobic exercise.

The mode of energy expenditure, not the total amount of energy expended, dictated the amount of fat loss; body weight was similar between the two groups. In other words, the low intensity group **lost more fat without a more negative energy balance**. In the Larson-Meyer energy deficit study, a 25% energy deficit from diet alone or from a combination of diet and exercise caused a similar effect on body weight but altered nutrient partitioning. Exercise tended to support muscle mass and enhance fat loss. Something very similar was seen in the Ballor aerobic exercise intensity study.

Growth hormone (GH) vs. insulin

1. GH makes you grow muscle and burn fat.

2. Insulin makes you grow adipose and store fat.

GH makes you grow muscle and burn fat; e.g., pubescent males, the GH studies cited above, the cjc-1295 studies cited above, etc.

1. **GH promotes food intake** to fuel muscle growth. Yes, adipose provides *some* of the fuel, which is why GH stimulates lipolysis, but cannot provide *all* of the fuel. So you eat more to:
    a. make up for the caloric difference, and
    b. provide an increased supply of the substrate amino acids.

2. **Insulin promotes food intake** to make you fat. Insulin, per se, does not stimulate appetite; e.g., type I diabetics have less/no insulin but are hyperphagic. However, insulin makes fat tissue grow. And growth requires increased food intake, just like with GH. It's just that with insulin the growth is fat tissue, whereas with GH the growth is muscle.

-While GH is under relatively non-controllable factors, for insulin just reduce carbs.

-You cannot easily (safely and legally) manipulate GH levels. It is easy to reduce insulin.

-GH is under relatively non-controllable factors, you cannot easily (safely and legally) manipulate GH levels.

-It is easy to reduce insulin, just reduce carbs.
-WSL

To recap:

-From Jorgensen's study, manipulation of the hormonal milieu via growth hormone supplementation is capable of reducing fat mass independent of energy balance.

-Two major effects of growth hormone are increased muscle hypertrophy and insulin antagonism. Increasing dietary protein and reducing carbohydrates recapitulates both of these effects.

-Ramsey's monkeys ate more food, gained lean mass, and lost body fat. In other words, they lost fat mass yet gained muscle despite being in a negative energy balance.

-Nutrient timing can promote fat loss and muscle hypertrophy independent from changes in energy balance. It's possible to significantly reduce fat mass by changing not only *what* you eat, but *when* you eat it.

-From Falutz's study (cjc-1295), we learned that minor shifts in hormone levels have the ability to completely remodel the metabolic landscape and induce profound changes in body composition independent of energy balance. It is frankly wrong to attribute 'getting fat' to a simple caloric surplus. The reverse is also true.

-From Buemann's study (ephedrine), the subjects selectively lost fat mass, and muscle was preserved. "A calorie is a calorie" and "eat less and move more" is wrong because these ideas refer to the regulation of *body weight*. The regulation of *fat mass* is critically more important, and in contrast with body weight, is not restricted to deviations in energy balance.

Chapter 15.
Exercise and appetite

Exercise makes you hungry

Exercise is one of the top two things people think of when the topic of weight loss comes up. Exercise increases overall fitness, improves cardiovascular health, and promotes a more positive well-being. One thing that exercise does not do, however, and this may come as a surprise, is cause weight loss. To be more specific, when someone initiates an exercise regimen, *without a specific dietary intervention*, long-term weight loss fails to occur in the majority of people. In brief, this is because the calorie deficit produced by exercising is too easily off-set by increased food intake. Sound familiar? Yes, this is very similar to what happens on a low calorie diet. Regardless of whether a calorie deficit is induced by exercise or a low fat diet, the body responds with increased hunger. So when a new exercise routine is begun, in the absence of a dietary intervention, this added hunger results in increased food intake, effectively negating the calorie deficit produced by exercise. Homeostasis.

There is one great example of this in the literature. In the late 1980's, Janssen and colleagues recruited a group of sedentary, healthy adults, and after a series of baseline measurements, started them on an 18-month marathon-training regimen *that did not include any dietary intervention* (Janssen, Graef et al. 1989). Training for a marathon is undoubtedly intense; thus, we can be certain that energy expenditure was increased relative to baseline. Over the course of the study, the subjects showed marked improvements in speed and endurance. This wasn't surprising, but it certainly provides confirmation that they really were working hard. The clincher? at the end of the study, the subjects actually ran in a real marathon!

Anyway, the intervention was specific to training only, there was no dietary advice. Lo and behold, after 18 months of a high-intensity endurance exercise program, body weight went largely unchanged. There were no significant reductions in body fat or increases in lean muscle tissue. Fortunately, although the authors refrained from giving any dietary advice, they did record food intake both at baseline and follow-up. Sure enough, the subjects ate more. A lot more. Predominantly carbohydrates. A standard, healthy, dinner of chicken, salad, and rice soon became chicken, salad, and 1.5 servings of rice... I am inclined to use this example because at the dinner table where I grew up, one piece of chicken would be prepared for each family member, and a large bowl of rice was placed in the center of the table; so if you were still hungry, you got more rice. The food intake data mentioned above support this possibility. The inability of 'exercise alone' to produce significant weight loss has been observed numerous times, with a variety of different exercise interventions. Quite simply, exercise 'builds up an appetite.'

Exercise really doesn't burn *that* many calories

It is not uncommon for people to exercise more if they know they are going to an event where large amounts of food are going to be served. Alternatively, some prefer to exercise after the party to burn-off the extra calories they just ate. Unfortunately, both are in for a surprise. A piece of cake may have around 400 kilocalories or so. To burn that off would require running 4 miles. Try running at about 6 miles an hour for 40 minutes. Or going for a two-hour hike. That amount of physical activity is enormous especially considering how easy it was eat that piece of cake. It might be practical to think you can exercise off the calories in a quarter-sized bite of chocolate, but not an entire dessert.

But isn't inactivity the cause of obesity? Obese people just aren't "burning off" everything they've eaten? Not really. For starters, researchers are practically polarized on the issue. One group believes that people get lazy, and this inactivity leads them to become obese. The other group believes that obese people are lazier, and that obesity causes inactivity. Both groups fail to acknowledge the critical role of food intake: 1. inactivity will not cause obesity unless it's accompanied by excessive food intake, and 2. excessive food intake can make an active person obese. These two observations suggest that food intake, as an independent variable, is necessary and sufficient to cause obesity. Furthermore, the fat storing effects of insulin implicate carbohydrates as a key component. Is it specific to sugars as opposed to fats or proteins? Yes, probably. Some observations: when Sumo wrestlers want to gain weight, they add carbohydrate-rich foods to their diet. Sumo wrestlers may not run marathons, but they are not necessarily "inactive." 2. To prepare the French delicacy foie gras (literally "fatty liver"), ducks are fed a very high-carbohydrate diet which increases fat deposition everywhere (especially in the liver). 3. Cattle are switched to a carb-rich diet of grains to increase the marbling (adipose) in their muscles. Overeating carbohydrates (which is relatively easy to do), in the absence of inactivity or laziness, is sufficient to induce obesity. Insulin, insulin resistance, and many of the usual suspects are probably involved (processed foods containing industrial trans fats, fructose, etc.). Thus, a poor diet is the cause of obesity. And a good diet can cure it.

Furthermore, the caloric expenditure of exercise is often overestimated. For example, take a healthy person with a VO_{2max} of 3 litres/min. If they exercise for **30 minutes at** 50% VO_{2max}:

$$3 \text{ L/min} * 50\% = 1.5 \text{ L/min}$$

$$1.5 \text{ L/min} * 30 \text{ min} = 45L \ O_2$$

$$45 \text{ L O2} \times 5 \text{ kcal/L} = 225 \text{ kcal}$$

225 kilocalories is less than 4 tablespoons of sugar. It's less than 2 tablespoons of butter. Doesn't 30 minutes of exercise seem like it should burn off more than a can of soda and a cookie?

Exercise is neither sufficient nor essential for weight loss

Diet + exercise is a great lifestyle choice that *will* improve your health, but it's not much more effective for weight loss than dieting + piano lessons.

This doesn't mean you shouldn't exercise.

Exercise benefits everyone. Fitness, regardless of bodyweight, is strongly associated with reduced all-cause mortality. With regard to the metabolic disturbances caused by a high glycemic index diet, exercise exerts a strong protective effect. Skeletal muscle is the major depository for blood glucose. Two distinct pathways operate in skeletal muscle to ensure glucose uptake can occur both in the 1) resting and 2) physically active states. The first pathway is necessary to clear excess dietary glucose and is activated by insulin. Insulin resistance affects this pathway and causes prolonged hyperglycemia, which may lead to chronic hyperinsulinemia and excessive fat accumulation, etc.

The second pathway is necessary to supplement working muscles with blood glucose for fuel and is activated directly by muscular contraction. Unlike insulin, however, the effects of muscle contraction are site specific; that is, glucose uptake is enhanced only in the contracting muscles.

In obesity, insulin- but not contraction-induced glucose uptake is impaired. In other words, obese muscles fail to respond to insulin as efficiently as lean muscles, but they respond perfectly well to contraction! Hyperglycemia and hyperinsulinemia are detrimental; an easy, safe, and extremely effective treatment [cure] would be for obese people to follow meals with a brief exercise session. It can be as little as a brisk walk, or climbing a flight of stairs. Although body weight is a much more important determinant of health, fitness also contributes. It *is* possible, as anyone who has tried to lose weight by exercise alone knows, to be 'fat but fit.'

What about someone on a low-carb diet? A low-carb diet is the single most effect preventative measure and cure for hyperglycemia and hyperinsulinemia, so would exercise provide any additional benefits to someone a low-carb diet? Yes. Although moderating glucose and insulin are two of the *major* benefits of exercise, they are not the *only* ones. Loss of skeletal muscle (sarcopenia, cachexia, low-calorie dieting, etc.) causes a host of

morbiditics and directly reduces quality of life.
Quality of life should never be underestimated.
Resistance, anaerobic, and strength training
improve the quantity, quality, and functional
capacity of skeletal muscle, which translates to
improved quality of life.

Lastly, exercise reduces stress! Thus,
preservation of lean muscle mass through exercise
has many benefits beyond glycemic control.

Exercise modality, calories, and appetite

For all conventional purposes, exercise
programs can be divided into two categories:
anaerobic and aerobic. Anaerobic training
promotes muscle growth and increases strength. It
is performed against resistance, usually with
weights. Aerobic exercise improves cardiovascular
fitness. Examples of aerobic exercise are running,
cycling, and swimming. During aerobic exercise
you are breathing heavy for an extended period of
time.

Anaerobic exercise is performed at a much
higher intensity than aerobic exercise. Exercise
intensity dictates fuel utilization: high intensity
anaerobic exercise (lifting weights) burns more
carbs (muscle glycogen, blood glucose) than fat

while low intensity aerobic exercise (running) burns more fat than carbs. Remember Ballor's exercise intensity study? jogging is lower intensity than running and therefore burns *proportionately* more fat (but less calories overall). Aerobic exercise intensity is determined by the rate of oxygen consumption. A fast runner may consume upwards of 1.5 litres of oxygen per minute while a slower runner may consume around 0.90 litres of oxygen per minute, for example.

Remember "respiratory quotient (RQ)" from **Chapter 2**? The RQ will be lower, reflecting greater fat oxidation, during a slow jog compared to a fast run. This is due to the differences in intensity. Even though a jogger burns proportionately more fat than a runner, the runner may burn more total fat because caloric expenditure is greater for running compared to jogging.

To compare 2-30 minute cardio sessions:

	L O_2 / min	RQ	kcal burned
run	1.5	0.87	250
jog	0.9	0.75	125

Fast running may use 60 % carbohydrates and 40 % fat, while slow jogging may use 30 % carbohydrates and 70 % fat. In other words, 40% of the fuel utilized during this theoretical fast run is derived from fat while 70% of the fuel utilized during the jog is derived from fat. When the total caloric expenditure is factored in, the jog burns *proportionately* more fat but the run burns more *total* fat.

	kcal burned		
	carbs	**fat**	**total**
run	150	100	250
jog	37	88	125

Given this information, you might think running is more efficient than jogging for fat loss. This is where it gets tricky. In the short term, i.e., *during* the exercise session, yes, running burns more fat than jogging. However, running breaks down more skeletal muscle than jogging. High intensity aerobic exercise burns both fat *and* muscle. Jogging or low-intensity aerobic exercise provides a great balance between cardiovascular fitness, fat burning, and muscle preservation (again, see Ballor's exercise intensity study above). In other words, I am saying that if you prefer aerobic to anaerobic exercise, run slower! ☺

Why is the muscle-burning effect of high intensity aerobic exercise important? For starters, time spent not exercising is significantly greater than time spent exercising. Therefore, even though exercise increases energy expenditure, the amount of calories expended while not exercising is much greater than those spent while exercising. Time spent not exercising is roughly 47 times longer than time spent exercising (30 minutes running vs. 23 ½ hours not running). Office work, sitting at a desk, grocery shopping, and sleeping are all lower intensity activities than running; therefore, compared to running, they burn proportionately more fat than carbs. And fat is burned by muscle. This, in a nutshell, is why jogging is superior to running for body composition. However, the optimal type of exercise is neither low nor high intensity aerobic exercise. Enter: anaerobic training.

Anaerobic, or "strength training" increases skeletal muscle mass. This directly improves strength, coordination, and quality of life. More importantly, having more skeletal muscle increases fat oxidation capacity. One reason for this is that having stronger muscles makes all activities easier, or lower intensity.   Lower intensity favors fat oxidation. In other words, to optimize the effects of exercise on fat burning, hit the weights.

Calories and fuel utilization

Weight training burns fewer calories, during the time spent exercising, than running or jogging. Although anaerobic exercise is more intense than aerobic exercise, the intensity comes in short bouts, i.e., only while you are lifting the weight. Most of the time in the weight room is spent resting in between sets or moving from one exercise to another. Due to its intrinsic high intensity, resistance exercise burns proportionately more carbs. This can be used to your advantage…

(FYI the following can be considered an adjunct to Nutrient Partitioning). During any type of exercise, *excess* carbs are burned first. Carbohydrate (glucose) is burned for harder or higher intensity exercise, and *all* types of exercise are hard at first. This has led some to believe that an exercise session should begin with anaerobic training, to burn off the excess carbs, and end with a cardio session, to optimize fat oxidation now that all the carbs are out of the way. Another way of thinking about this is that: first anaerobic exercise depletes glycogen, then the body has no choice but to rely of fat oxidation to fuel the aerobic exercise. This may be true, but in reality, however, the difference is not very robust. That doesn't mean you shouldn't train this way. Cardio makes you sweat. Do aerobic exercise after lifting weights if you don't want to walk around the gym all sweaty (and also there's a slight possibility it may be modestly more effective for fat loss). Moreover, there is one potentially legitimate reason to do strength training first: aerobic training is tiring; it will decrease the intensity of a subsequent resistance training bout. Strength training does little to your aerobic capacity, so aerobic exercise performance won't be diminished by a prior strength training session.

Conclusion: Lift heavy weights daily and take a few brisk walks or jogs every week. If there is a history of heart disease, low-intensity aerobic exercise should be performed every day or as much as possible. If you have any conditions associated with elevated blood glucose (hyperglycemia, pre-diabetes, type II diabetes mellitus, etc.), perform some sort of physical activity after each meal.

Exercise performance and diet

This section has little to do with calories, appetite, and obesity. It is about the role of diet in exercise and athletic performance.

Eating a low carbohydrate diet will reduce the body's glucose load. For athletes, this means reduced glycogen storage. As discussed above, glycogen and glucose are required for high intensity activities. The relationship between this and athletic performance has been examined scientifically in some very interesting experiments.

An early study by Phinney and colleagues set out to test the extremes (Phinney, Bistrian et al. 1983). In this experiment, they recruited endurance-trained athletes. In many instances, the use of trained athletes is disadvantageous because most of us are not trained athletes. Sedentary people will not respond to an exercise intervention the same way a trained athlete will. One advantage of using trained athletes, on the other hand, is there is no learning curve. If you bring in a sedentary subject and take measurements before and after an exercise routine, they are going to show many great improvements in strength and endurance. However, much of this is due to the learning curve. In other words, there are neural adaptations to exercise. They may not be getting stronger, per se, but they will be able to lift heavier weight because gradually during the intervention they will learn how to perform the exercise better or more efficiently. Thus, they will be stronger not because of increased strength but because of neural adaptation. This is OK in some studies, if that is the focus, but not in all studies.

In Phinney's study the athletes were cyclists and they were given a normal diet for a week to take baseline measurements and then an isocaloric very low carbohydrate diet for over three weeks. A major strength of this study is that it lasted longer than three weeks. Three weeks is too short for a diet study, but not for the question being asked in this particular exercise study. More specifically, athletes require a period of time to adapt to new diets; given the essential role of glycogen in athletic performance, this is especially true for low carbohydrate diets. And this adaptation takes a few weeks. Therefore, by the time final measurements are made, we can be sure that the results are not an artefact of the adaptation (like what is seen when sedentary people are first put on an exercise program).

Another strength is that the study was done on subjects who were in weight maintenance. Weight loss or being in a weight-reduced state alters fuel utilization considerably. Although gaining information about those conditions is important, they are asking different questions. This study was designed to test the effect of a specific diet on exercise performance; weight loss would interfere with this so food intake was tailored to keep all the participants weight-stable. The diets were as follows:

	~3400 kcal / day		
	protein	CHO	fat
control	16%	56%	28%
ketogenic	16%	1%	82%

Note the almost complete absence of carbohydrates in the ketogenic diet; this will rapidly reduce muscle glycogen and promote a high level of lipolysis and fat oxidation.

These were elite cyclists, whose training included riding upwards of 300 miles per week. This training was continued throughout the study. VO_{2max} testing consists of riding a stationary cycle pretty fast, against resistance, and the speed and/or resistance progressively increase until the athlete can't keep up (or when their RQ exceeds 1, see below). **VO_{2max}, a measure of maximal athletic performance, was approximately 5 litres per minute and was not affected by a very low carbohydrate diet.**

Respiratory quotient (RQ) during the VO_{2max} was 1.04 at baseline. In general, an RQ value greater than 1 means a mistake was made. This does not usually happen. Recall, respiratory quotient is the ratio of carbon dioxide produced divided by the amount of oxygen consumed. When performing very high intensity work, carbon dioxide is produced as a byproduct of the work being performed, and oxygen consumption increases accordingly. However, as intensity gets *really* high, oxygen consumption eventually plateaus; the athlete simply cannot breathe any faster. But CO_2 production still increases due to continued fuel oxidation and acid-base imbalances. Under these conditions RQ will exceed 1. Interestingly, however, RQ was only 0.90 on the ketogenic diet. A lower RQ is expected on a ketogenic diet, which reflects a greater reliance on fat oxidation. But during VO_{2max} testing, the high intensity is thought to require glucose oxidation… This doesn't mean that they were working less hard, because their VO_{2max} was the same. It means they adapted. **After the adaptation period their body was able to achieve the <u>same degree of intensity </u>with less glucose oxidation and more fat oxidation.** Interesting.

Next they tested endurance. Endurance testing consists of cycling at a power equivalent to 65% of VO_{2max} until exhaustion. VO_{2max} was 5 litres per minute, so the researchers set the endurance exercise to a level where the athletes would be consuming oxygen at a rate of approximately 3.2 litres per minute. **Time to exhaustion at 65% VO_{2max} was 147 minutes at baseline and, similar to the VO_{2max}, was unaffected by a very low carbohydrate diet.** RQ during the endurance testing at baseline was 0.83. As expected, this was much lower than RQ during VO_{2max} at baseline (1.04) because it was performed at a much lower intensity. This is because when exercising at a lower intensity, fat oxidation increases, glucose oxidation decreases, and therefore RQ goes down. When they were exercising at 100% VO_{2max}, the high reliance on glucose oxidation produced an RQ of 1.04. When exercising at 65% VO_{2max}, increased fat oxidation produced an RQ of 0.83. During the ketogenic diet, however, RQ was only 0.72. They were riding at the same intensity for the control and ketogenic diet periods (VO_2 = 3.2 litres per minute), but after adaptation they were able to produce more power burning fat than before. More importantly, total power (VO_{2max}) and endurance (time to exhaustion), arguably the two most important determinants of athletic performance, were not affected by a very low carbohydrate diet. *This* is adaptation. In other words, given a sufficient adaptation period ($\sim$ 3-4 weeks in this case), exercise performance will not suffer because of insufficient dietary carbohydrates.

What about muscle glycogen levels? Glycogen levels are, in part, controlled by dietary carbohydrates and physical activity levels. After a carbohydrate-free diet, muscle glycogen declined from 143 to 76 (millimoles of glycosyl units per kilogram of muscle), confirming the importance of dietary carbohydrates in maintaining muscle glycogen content. During the endurance tests on the control diet, muscle glycogen declined from 143 to 53, a net decrease of 90. After the ketogenic diet, however, muscle glycogen declined from 76 to 56, a net decrease of 20. 90 versus 20: 90 is significantly greater than 20, which confirms the RQ data that showed greater carbohydrate oxidation on the control diet. Less muscle glycogen utilization during the ketogenic diet is also confirmed by the lower RQ which reflects increased fat oxidation. The body adapts, and these researchers took meticulous care in capturing the most important measurements in order to empirically quantify this adaptation. Of course, there are hundreds of diets, exercise variations, and subject populations that would be interesting to test. And just because adaptation occurred in this population doesn't mean that it will occur in every population. However, this study is important because it demonstrates that adaptation *can* and *does* happen.

As stated above, the body generally doesn't manifest the same amount of power from oxidizing different nutrients. This might be considered another angle supporting that all calories are not created equal. *And* the fuel requirements for a set amount of power output can change! Regardless of any theorized metabolic advantage of one diet or another, it is clear that all calories are quite simply not the same. The *additional energy expenditure for protein turnover and gluconeogenesis on a high protein diet*, and the *amount of power generated from oxidizing glucose compared to fat* are two examples suggesting all calories are not the same.

The Phinney study is not an isolated case. Vogt and colleagues did a similar study where they fed 11 athletes either a 17% fat or a 53% fat diet for 5 weeks (Vogt, Puntschart et al. 2003). Although the diet was not ketogenic as in Phinney's study, there was still a large reduction in carbohydrate intake in the high fat group (31% vs. 68% in the high and low fat groups, respectively). Importantly, the study lasted long enough for the athletes to adapt to the diet. This study was done in a crossover design, which is one of the strongest study designs for human intervention trials. A simple crossover study would be, for example, two subjects, Jake and Andrew, and two treatments: A and B. At first, Jake receives treatment A while Andrew receives treatment B. Then after a predetermined 'washout' period, Jake receives treatment B and Andrew receives treatment A.

This type of study design automatically controls for virtually all potential confounding factors because the response of Jake to treatment A is not only compared to Andrew on treatment B, it is also compared to Jake on treatment B. It allows for a very clear examination of the interventions.

The study results: in brief, there were no changes in body weight or body composition, although as expected, the high fat [low carb] group had modestly lower muscle glycogen (488 vs. 534 mmoles/kg) and significantly increased intramyocellular lipids (0.69% vs. 1.54%). Intramyocellular lipids are triacylglycerol or fat stores inside of muscle. In athletes, these fat stores are used for energy during exercise. **VO_{2max} was 64 mL/min*kg and unaffected by diet**; further confirming that a high fat low carb diet does not impair an athlete's maximal power output. Similarly, **total power output during an ultra-high intensity 20-minute "all-out" cycling was the same in both groups (~298 watts).** Maximum intensity and power were unaffected by diet, and both tests were performed on a cycle. However, the researchers also measured performance in a completely different paradigm: how long it took them to run a half-marathon (~13 miles). As opposed to generating power and intensity, running a half-marathon requires endurance and a high aerobic capacity. They found that it took both groups 80 minutes. **Endurance was unaffected by a low carb high fat diet.** In other words, after a significant adaptation period, virtually every measure of athletic performance was similar when the high fat group cut their carb intake by more than half. This is definitely against the grain of current thought in many athletic circles, but the most important factor is a proper adaptation period.

The researchers also performed a graded submaximal exercise test, where a battery of measurements are made while the subjects are cycling at various percentages of their maximum work output "W_{max}" (which was 298 watts in both groups). For example, at 20% W_{max}, absolute work was 76 watts while at 75% W_{max}, absolute work was 283 watts. The absolute work performed was the same in both groups because W_{max} was the same. In both groups, respiratory quotient was lower during low intensity compared to high intensity work. In the low fat group, working at 20% W_{max} produced a respiratory quotient of 0.97 while working at 75% W_{max} produced a respiratory quotient of 1.05. Harder work requires more glucose oxidation, which produces a higher respiratory quotient. The intensity at which an athlete's respiratory quotient becomes greater than one is an important biomarker that they are officially working hard.

For the high fat group, respiratory quotient at 20% W_{max} was significantly lower than the low fat group, 0.89, reflecting a greater reliance of fat oxidation during low intensity work. At 75% W_{max}, respiratory quotient became 1.0. Two interesting points: 1) the difference in respiratory quotient between the high and low fat groups was much bigger during low intensity exercise. This is because the fuel requirements for low intensity work are more flexible than for high intensity work. If your team is up against a significantly less skillful opponent, you can put in whatever players you want. But if your team is playing a great team, you don't have so much flexibility in deciding who will play; in order to win you have to play your best players. During high intensity exercise, the difference in respiratory quotient between the groups is much smaller than low intensity exercise because the higher power output absolutely requires greater glucose oxidation rates. The interesting finding was that at every intensity level, respiratory quotient was lower for the high fat group, and their respiratory quotient even crossed

1 at a higher level of absolute work. In other words, when both groups were exercising at maximum intensity (which was the same in both groups), those fed the high fat diet seemed to be working relatively less hard. Their respiratory quotient didn't exceed 1 until they were working at over 75% W_{max}, while the low fat group's respiratory quotient exceeded 1 at 60%. Although there is no clear measurement for this, this finding suggests that the high fat group was, in some regard, generating a higher power output more efficiently. Interesting indeed.

In sum, a calorie is not a calorie. Two grams of glucose or one gram of fat may produce similar heat in a bomb calorimeter, but this doesn't translate into how they are treated by the body. The body uses carbohydrates for different things than it does protein and fats, and each of these processes have different energy requirements and function at different levels of efficiency.

Fatigue and muscle glycogen

It is currently thought amongst athletes and fitness enthusiasts that adequate muscle glycogen levels are required for optimal performance.

However, this is simply not true and half of the evidence has already been described in this book.

To recap:

-Phinney's cyclists: 4 weeks of a ketogenic very low carb diet reduced muscle glycogen levels but had no effect on VO_{2max} and time to exhaustion at 65% $VO2_{max}$.

-Vogt's athletes: 5 weeks of a low carb diet reduced muscle glycogen levels but had no effect on VO_{2max}, 20-minute all-out cycling power output, or the time it took to run a half-marathon.

These two studies show that reduced muscle glycogen levels have no effect on the most validated and important scientific measurements of athletic performance. Speed, power, and endurance were all maintained in subjects consuming carbohydrate-restricted diets.

Technically, it was not only muscle glycogen levels that were altered in those two studies; diet was altered also. So it is possible, albeit somewhat abstract, that lower glycogen levels do indeed reduce performance, but some other manifestation of the low-carb diet was intrinsically ergogenic which masked the effects of lower glycogen. This could be tested in two ways: 1) put athletes on a low-carb diet then artificially increase their muscle glycogen levels and see if performance improves; and 2) take athletes on a mixed diet then reduce their muscle glycogen levels and see if performance declines. Option #1 is kind-of-impossible because any treatment to increase muscle glycogen would include carbohydrates and insulin which would completely nullify their low-carb status.

One remarkable study, one of my favorite exercise studies of all time, indirectly addressed Option #2 (Coyle, Coggan et al. 1986). In their first experiment, glycogen utilization was measured following 105 minutes of exercise at 71.4% VO_{2max} with or without carbohydrate supplementation. Since these were endurance-trained cyclists, this level of intensity is probably at or just below their lactate threshold (which occurs at ~75% in athletes and 55% in non-athletes). VO_{2max} was measured to be ~4.72 L/min (69.8 mL/kg*min), which is rather high (confirming that these were indeed well-trained athletes, and they were good). The carbohydrate supplementation was given to displace glycogen utilization; in this group, most of the glucose used to fuel exercise would come from blood glucose instead of muscle glycogen. Furthermore, the study was designed as a crossover study which, as stated above, controls for virtually all conceivable confounding variables by testing all the subjects under both conditions on separate occasions. It was also double blind and placebo-controlled, which means that the subjects not receiving carbohydrate supplementation instead drank an artificially sweetened beverage that tasted exactly like the carbohydrate drink, and neither the investigators nor the subjects knew which one they were getting (so it couldn't be biased in any way). The carbohydrate supplement consisted of a glucose dose of 0.4mg/kg, which worked to be ~27.04 grams of glucose in 270mL ingested every 20 minutes for the duration of the experiment. Muscle glycogen content was ~119 mmoles/kg at baseline and declined to ~43 mmoles/kg after 105 minutes *in both groups.* Muscle glycogen declined just as much in the carbohydrate group, who had consumed a total of 135.2 grams of glucose during the exercise session, as it did in the placebo group. These findings suggest that muscle glycogen, not blood glucose, is the primary fuel during *sub-exhaustion* exercise. In other words, the glucose from their carbohydrate beverage did not displace muscle glycogen utilization. However, this also meant that the experiment didn't work; the carbohydrate beverage was supposed to spare muscle glycogen, but it didn't. The type of exercise dictated fuel preference, not fuel availability (during *sub-exhaustion* exercise). So the investigators performed a second experiment where the subjects were asked to cycle until exhaustion. For endurance-trained cyclists, this is much, much longer. The researchers wanted to see what would happen when glycogen stores were all used up.

In the second experiment, the same general procedure was performed but the subjects cycled until they were completely fatigued. The placebo group fatigued at 3 hours while the carbohydrate group fatigued at 4 hours, by which time they had ingested ~324 grams or ~1,300 kilocalories of glucose. Given that their VO_{2max} was 4.71 L/min and they were exercising at 71.4%, their VO_2 during exercise would have been 3.37 L/min. If we use the rough estimate of 5 kcal for the energetic value for a litre of O_2, then they were expending 16.85 kcal / min. After 3 or 4 hours, the total expenditure would have been ~3,033 and 4,044 kcal in the placebo and carbohydrate groups, respectively (that is a LOT of calories).

Here is where the truly interesting data arose. First, respiratory quotient in the placebo group was around 0.85, confirming a relatively high glucose oxidation during the first 2 hours of their session. After that, respiratory quotient began to decline reflecting increased fat oxidation (which as stated above, happens with increased exercise duration), until they fatigued at three hours. The drop in respiratory quotient was most likely due to reduced glucose availability. From the first experiment, we know muscle glycogen is the preferred fuel for this type of exercise, and we also know that after 1 hour and 45 minutes muscle glycogen is reduced to around 40 mmoles/kg (in both groups). But respiratory quotient remained high in the carbohydrate supplemented group for the entire 4 hours, which would suggest that they were still burning glucose. The placebo group still was still burning muscle glycogen when they became exhausted; in other words, they reached fatigue *before* they ran out of glycogen. After 3 and a half hours, muscle glycogen was no longer providing fuel for the carbohydrate supplemented group, suggesting that their glucose supply was coming directly from the bloodstream; in other words, they were still exercising long *after* exhausting their glycogen supply. In both cases, glucose availability, not muscle glycogen levels, determined fatigue. Elevated blood glucose, as in the carbohydrate supplemented group, does not spare muscle glycogen; lower blood glucose, as in the placebo group (during the third and final hour of their ride), does not accelerate muscle glycogen degradation. Between hours 3 and 4, cycling in the carbohydrate supplemented group was predominantly fueled by blood glucose, not muscle glycogen.

Athletes on a ketogenic diet can run as far and fast as those on a mixed diet, but they have lower glycogen levels *and* have no dietary glucose intake. How do they maintain high performance with limited glucose availability? The results of Coyle would suggest that glucose availability, regardless of its form, is important for optimal performance. The results of Phinney and Vogt suggest that carbohydrates aren't required for optimal performance. Furthermore, the RQ data from both studies indicate that fat oxidation can in fact fuel high performance. Carbohydrate restriction offers a wide range of health benefits to the general population and especially to obese or overweight people. Since it apparently has no effect on performance, should athletes switch to low-carb diets?

Appendix

Appendix A. Population-specific macronutrient intake

Relative caloric contribution of carbohydrates, fat, and protein in various diets around the world (just a collection from mixed references, feel free to add some more!)

	carbs	fat	protein
low-carb	10%	60%	30%
Greek	41%	40%	19%
Western	55%	30%	15%
Kitavan	70%	20%	10%
Japan	79%	8%	13%
Okinawa	85%	6%	9%

Appendix B. Work and power conversions

	kJ / min	kcal / min	kg*m/min	Watts (J/s)
kJ / min	1.0	0.2389	0.000102	16.667
kcal / min	4.186	1.0	426.85	0
kg*m/min	6.16	0.00234	1.0	0.163
Watts (J/s)	0.06	0.01433	6.118	1.0

Conversions, et al.

- $VO_2 = ml/(kg \times min) = (L/min \times 1000) / BM \ (kg)$
- VO_2 Reserve $= (VO_{2max} - \text{resting } VO_2)$
- $1 \ MET = 3.5 \ ml/ \ (kg \times min)$
- $1 \ L$ of O_2 consumed $= 5 \ kcal$
- 1 lb. of fat $= 3500 \ kcal$
- Watts $=$ work rate $(kg/m \times min) \div 6.12$
- $1 \ kg = 2.2046 \ lbs \ (kg = lbs \div 2.2046)$
- $1 \ mph = 26.8 \ m/min \ (mph \times 26.8 = m/min)$
- $1 \ kph = 16.67 \ m/min \ (kph / 0.06 = m/min)$
- $1 \ in = 0.0254 \ m \ (0.0254 \times in = m)$

Kcal $/ \ L \ O_2 \approx RQ + 4$

Power (watts) $=$ work / time
$\qquad = $ (force $\times$ distance) / time

1Watt$= 6.12 \ (kg \times m) \ /min$

1 meter $= 3.28$ feet
1 mile $= 5,280$ feet $= 1.62 \ km$

1 mph $= 26.8$ meters / min $= 1.62 \ km/h$

1 km/h $= 0.62$ mph

VO2 (mL/ [kg $\times$ min]) $\times \ 5 \ = $ kcal / min

Appendix C. Energy: per gram vs. per litre O_2

	kcal/g	kcal/L O_2
carbs	4	5.05
protein	4	4.5
fat	9	4.7

RQ	**fuel %**		**kcal / L O_2**
	glucose	**fat**	
0.7	0%	100%	4.686
0.75	15%	85%	4.739
0.8	32%	68%	4.801
0.85	49%	51%	4.862
0.9	**66%**	**34%**	**4.924**
0.95	83%	17%	4.985
1	100%	0%	5.047

On average: 1 litre $O_2 \approx 5$ kcal. For a more precise estimation: 1 litre $O_2 \approx 4 + RQ$.

Examples I. Fuels burned during a 30 minute exercise session

Measured:

Exercise VO_2:	2.15 L/min
RQ:	0.90

4.924 kcal / L O_2 x 2.15 L / min = 10.59 kcal/min

10.59 kcal/min x 30 min = 318 kcal

318 kcal x 66% glucose = 210 kcal glucose

318 kcal x 34% fat = 108 kcal fat

Examples II.

Average VO2max ≈ 46.7 mL O_2 / (kg x min)

                                ≈ 3.5 mL O_2 / min

The average person would reach this by running at

        ≈ 11.2 km/hr

        ≈ 7 mph

Running a mile in 8 minutes 34 seconds

1 MET = 3.5 mL O_2 / (kg x min)

1 MET = 1 kcal / (kg x hr)

Lactate threshold:

        55% VO_{2max} in untrained individuals

        75% VO_{2max} in athletes

Oxygen consumption while going uphill:

1.8 mL O_2 / kg   x   meters/min   x   grade

Appendix D. RQ anomalies

RQ = CO_2 produced / O_2 consumed

RQ > 1
De novo lipogenesis, or converting carbs into fat (requires high carbohydrate intake and high insulin levels). RQ > 1 because glucose contains much more oxygen than fat. This oxygen is released as CO_2, driving up the numerator in the RQ equation.

During exhaustive exercise.
RQ > 1 because of excess "non-metabolic" CO_2 production. The source of this CO_2 is the blood bicarbonate buffering system. This CO_2 arises during by the acidotic conditions produced during exhaustive exercise.

RQ < 1
Gluconeogenesis, or converting other fuels into glucose. RQ < 1 because oxygen must be added to other fuels to make glucose, driving up the denominator in the RQ equation.

Appendix E. Phenotypes of mice with altered 11β-HSD1 expression

11β-HSD1	BW	Food intake	VAT	insulin sensitivity	overall health
adipose overexpression	↑	↑	↑	↓↓	bad
liver overexpression	↔		↔	↓	inter-mediate
knockout	↓	↑	↓	↑↑	good

Index

320

William Castelli, 108
work, 289

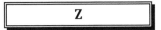

Bibliography

Anselmi, C. V., A. Malovini, et al. (2009). "Association of the FOXO3A locus with extreme longevity in a southern Italian centenarian study." Rejuvenation Res **12**(2): 95-104.

Balkau, B., M. Shipley, et al. (1998). "High blood glucose concentration is a risk factor for mortality in middle-aged nondiabetic men. 20-year follow-up in the Whitehall Study, the Paris Prospective Study, and the Helsinki Policemen Study." Diabetes Care **21**(3): 360-367.

Ballor, D. L., J. P. McCarthy, et al. (1990). "Exercise intensity does not affect the composition of diet- and exercise-induced body mass loss." Am J Clin Nutr **51**(2): 142-146.

Baur, J. A., K. J. Pearson, et al. (2006). "Resveratrol improves health and survival of mice on a high-calorie diet." Nature **444**(7117): 337-342.

Bluher, M., B. B. Kahn, et al. (2003). "Extended longevity in mice lacking the insulin receptor in adipose tissue." Science **299**(5606): 572-574.

Bluher, M., M. D. Michael, et al. (2002). "Adipose tissue selective insulin receptor knockout protects against obesity and obesity-related glucose intolerance." Dev Cell **3**(1): 25-38.

Borst, S. E., C. F. Conover, et al. (2005). "Association of resistin with visceral fat and muscle insulin resistance." Cytokine **32**(1): 39-44.

Buemann, B., P. Marckmann, et al. (1994). "The effect of ephedrine plus caffeine on plasma lipids and lipoproteins during a 4.2 MJ/day diet." Int J Obes Relat Metab Disord **18**(5): 329-332.

Burr, M. L., A. M. Fehily, et al. (1989). "Effects of changes in fat, fish, and fibre intakes on death and myocardial reinfarction: diet and reinfarction trial (DART)." Lancet **2**(8666): 757-761.

Castelli, W. P. (1992). "Concerning the possibility of a nut." Arch Intern Med **152**(7): 1371-1372.

Chiasson, J. L., R. G. Josse, et al. (2003). "Acarbose treatment and the risk of cardiovascular disease and hypertension in patients with impaired glucose tolerance: the STOP-NIDDM trial." JAMA **290**(4): 486-494.

Coyle, E. F., A. R. Coggan, et al. (1986). "Muscle glycogen utilization during prolonged strenuous exercise when fed carbohydrate." J Appl Physiol **61**(1): 165-172.

Cribb, P. J. and A. Hayes (2006). "Effects of supplement timing and resistance exercise on skeletal muscle hypertrophy." Med Sci Sports Exerc **38**(11): 1918-1925.

Crowe, M. J., J. N. Weatherson, et al. (2006). "Effects of dietary leucine supplementation on exercise performance." Eur J Appl Physiol **97**(6): 664-672.

Diaz, E. O., A. M. Prentice, et al. (1992). "Metabolic response to experimental overfeeding in lean and overweight healthy volunteers." Am J Clin Nutr **56**(4): 641-655.

Duda, M. K., K. M. O'Shea, et al. (2009). "Fish oil, but not flaxseed oil, decreases inflammation and prevents pressure overload-induced cardiac dysfunction." Cardiovasc Res **81**(2): 319-327.

Due, A., S. Toubro, et al. (2004). "Effect of normal-fat diets, either medium or high in protein, on body weight in overweight subjects: a randomised 1-year trial." Int J Obes Relat Metab Disord **28**(10): 1283-1290.

Esmarck, B., J. L. Andersen, et al. (2001). "Timing of postexercise protein intake is important for muscle hypertrophy with resistance training in elderly humans." J Physiol **535**(Pt 1): 301-311.

Falutz, J., S. Allas, et al. (2005). "A placebo-controlled, dose-ranging study of a growth hormone releasing factor in HIV-infected patients with abdominal fat accumulation." AIDS **19**(12): 1279-1287.

Flachsbart, F., A. Caliebe, et al. (2009). "Association of FOXO3A variation with human longevity confirmed in German centenarians." Proc Natl Acad Sci U S A **106**(8): 2700-2705.

Gabriely, I., X. H. Ma, et al. (2002). "Removal of visceral fat prevents insulin resistance and glucose intolerance of aging: an adipokine-mediated process?" Diabetes **51**(10): 2951-2958.

Gerstein, H. C., M. E. Miller, et al. (2008). "Effects of intensive glucose lowering in type 2 diabetes." N Engl J Med **358**(24): 2545-2559.

Grey, N. and D. M. Kipnis (1971). "Effect of diet composition on the hyperinsulinemia of obesity." N Engl J Med **285**(15): 827-831.

Griffin, M. E., A. Feder, et al. (2001). "Lipoatrophy associated with lispro insulin in insulin pump therapy: an old complication, a new cause?" Diabetes Care **24**(1): 174.

Harrison, D. E., J. R. Archer, et al. (1984). "Effects of food restriction on aging: separation of food intake and adiposity." Proc Natl Acad Sci U S A **81**(6): 1835-1838.

Hauswirth, C. B., M. R. Scheeder, et al. (2004). "High omega-3 fatty acid content in alpine cheese: the basis for an alpine paradox." Circulation **109**(1): 103-107.

Horton, T. J., H. Drougas, et al. (1995). "Fat and carbohydrate overfeeding in humans: different effects on energy storage." Am J Clin Nutr **62**(1): 19-29.

Howard, B. V., J. E. Manson, et al. (2006). "Low-fat dietary pattern and weight change over 7 years: the Women's Health Initiative Dietary Modification Trial." JAMA **295**(1): 39-49.

Hu, F. B., M. J. Stampfer, et al. (1997). "Dietary fat intake and the risk of coronary heart disease in women." N Engl J Med **337**(21): 1491-1499.

Janssen, G. M., C. J. Graef, et al. (1989). "Food intake and body composition in novice athletes during a training period to run a marathon." Int J Sports Med **10 Suppl 1**: S17-21.

Johnson, P. R., J. S. Stern, et al. (1997). "Longevity in obese and lean male and female rats of the Zucker strain: prevention of hyperphagia." Am J Clin Nutr **66**(4): 890-903.

Jonsson, T., S. Olsson, et al. (2005). "Agrarian diet and diseases of affluence--do evolutionary novel dietary lectins cause leptin resistance?" BMC Endocr Disord **5**: 10.

Jorgensen, A. P., K. J. Fougner, et al. (2011). "Favorable long-term effects of growth hormone replacement therapy on quality of life, bone metabolism, body composition and lipid levels in patients with adult-onset growth hormone deficiency." Growth Horm IGF Res.

Kavanagh, K., K. L. Jones, et al. (2007). "Trans fat diet induces abdominal obesity and changes in insulin sensitivity in monkeys." Obesity (Silver Spring) **15**(7): 1675-1684.

Klein, S., L. Fontana, et al. (2004). "Absence of an effect of liposuction on insulin action and risk factors for coronary heart disease." N Engl J Med **350**(25): 2549-2557.

Knatterud, G. L., C. R. Klimt, et al. (1978). "Effects of hypoglycemic agents on vascular complications in patients with adult-onset diabetes. VII. Mortality and selected nonfatal events with insulin treatment." JAMA **240**(1): 37-42.

Knott, S. A., L. J. Cummins, et al. (2010). "Feed efficiency and body composition are related to cortisol response to adrenocorticotropin hormone and insulin-induced hypoglycemia in rams." Domest Anim Endocrinol **39**(2): 137-146.

Kolotkin, R. L., R. D. Crosby, et al. (2009). "Two-year changes in health-related quality of life in gastric bypass patients compared with severely obese controls." Surg Obes Relat Dis **5**(2): 250-256.

Larsen, T. M., S. M. Dalskov, et al. (2010). "Diets with high or low protein content and glycemic index for weight-loss maintenance." N Engl J Med **363**(22): 2102-2113.

Larson-Meyer, D. E., L. K. Heilbronn, et al. (2006). "Effect of calorie restriction with or without exercise on insulin sensitivity, beta-cell function, fat cell size, and ectopic lipid in overweight subjects." Diabetes Care **29**(6): 1337-1344.

Lee, C., L. R. Giles, et al. (2005). "The effect of active immunization against adrenocorticotropic hormone on cortisol, beta-endorphin, vocalization, and growth in pigs." J Anim Sci **83**(10): 2372-2379.

Li, X., M. B. Cope, et al. (2010). "Mild calorie restriction induces fat accumulation in female C57BL/6J mice." Obesity (Silver Spring) **18**(3): 456-462.

Li, Y., W. J. Wang, et al. (2009). "Genetic association of FOXO1A and FOXO3A with longevity trait in Han Chinese populations." Hum Mol Genet **18**(24): 4897-4904.

Lindeberg, S., M. Eliasson, et al. (1999). "Low serum insulin in traditional Pacific Islanders--the Kitava Study." Metabolism **48**(10): 1216-1219.

Lindeberg, S., P. Nilsson-Ehle, et al. (1994). "Cardiovascular risk factors in a Melanesian population apparently free from stroke and ischaemic heart disease: the Kitava study." J Intern Med **236**(3): 331-340.

Lustig, R. H. (2008). "Which comes first? The obesity or the insulin? The behavior or the biochemistry?" J Pediatr **152**(5): 601-602.

Marchioli, R. (1999). "[Results of GISSI Prevenzione: diet, drugs, and cardiovascular risk. Researchers of GISSI Prevenzione]." Cardiologia **44 Suppl 1**(Pt 2): 745-746.

Masuzaki, H., J. Paterson, et al. (2001). "A transgenic model of visceral obesity and the metabolic syndrome." Science **294**(5549): 2166-2170.

McDevitt, R. M., S. D. Poppitt, et al. (2000). "Macronutrient disposal during controlled overfeeding with glucose, fructose, sucrose, or

fat in lean and obese women." Am J Clin Nutr
72(2): 369-377.

Mitchell, J. E., K. L. Lancaster, et al. (2001). "Long-term
follow-up of patients' status after gastric
bypass." Obes Surg 11(4): 464-468.

Morton, N. M., J. M. Paterson, et al. (2004). "Novel
adipose tissue-mediated resistance to diet-
induced visceral obesity in 11 beta-
hydroxysteroid dehydrogenase type 1-deficient
mice." Diabetes 53(4): 931-938.

Mozaffarian, D., E. B. Rimm, et al. (2004). "Dietary fats,
carbohydrate, and progression of coronary
atherosclerosis in postmenopausal women."
Am J Clin Nutr 80(5): 1175-1184.

Oppert, J. M., A. Nadeau, et al. (1995). "Plasma glucose,
insulin, and glucagon before and after long-
term overfeeding in identical twins."
Metabolism 44(1): 96-105.

Pawlikowska, L., D. Hu, et al. (2009). "Association of
common genetic variation in the insulin/IGF1
signaling pathway with human longevity." Aging
Cell 8(4): 460-472.

Phinney, S. D., B. R. Bistrian, et al. (1983). "The human
metabolic response to chronic ketosis without
caloric restriction: preservation of submaximal
exercise capability with reduced carbohydrate
oxidation." Metabolism 32(8): 769-776.

Rahmadi, A., N. Steiner, et al. (2011). "Review:
Advanced glycation endproducts as
gerontotoxins and biomarkers for carbonyl-
based degenerative processes in Alzheimer's
disease." Clin Chem Lab Med.

Ramsey, J. J., R. J. Colman, et al. (2000). "Dietary
restriction and aging in rhesus monkeys: the

University of Wisconsin study." Exp Gerontol
35(9-10): 1131-1149.

Ramsey, J. J., R. J. Colman, et al. (1998). "Energy
expenditure, body composition, and glucose
metabolism in lean and obese rhesus monkeys
treated with ephedrine and caffeine." Am J Clin
Nutr **68**(1): 42-51.

Richard, J. L. (1987). "[Coronary risk factors. The French
paradox]." Arch Mal Coeur Vaiss **80 Spec No**:
17-21.

Rosenbaum, M., R. Goldsmith, et al. (2005). "Low-dose
leptin reverses skeletal muscle, autonomic, and
neuroendocrine adaptations to maintenance of
reduced weight." J Clin Invest **115**(12): 3579-
3586.

Roust, L. R., K. D. Hammel, et al. (1994). "Effects of
isoenergetic, low-fat diets on energy
metabolism in lean and obese women." Am J
Clin Nutr **60**(4): 470-475.

Salomon, F., R. C. Cuneo, et al. (1989). "The effects of
treatment with recombinant human growth
hormone on body composition and metabolism
in adults with growth hormone deficiency." N
Engl J Med **321**(26): 1797-1803.

Serra-Majem, L., L. Ribas, et al. (1995). "How could
changes in diet explain changes in coronary
heart disease mortality in Spain? The Spanish
paradox." Am J Clin Nutr **61**(6 Suppl): 1351S-
1359S.

Simopoulos, A. P. (2001). "Evolutionary aspects of diet
and essential fatty acids." World Rev Nutr Diet
88: 18-27.

Stern, L., N. Iqbal, et al. (2004). "The effects of low-
carbohydrate versus conventional weight loss

diets in severely obese adults: one-year follow-up of a randomized trial." <u>Ann Intern Med</u> **140**(10): 778-785.

Studer, M., M. Briel, et al. (2005). "Effect of different antilipidemic agents and diets on mortality: a systematic review." <u>Arch Intern Med</u> **165**(7): 725-730.

Tinker, L. F., D. E. Bonds, et al. (2008). "Low-fat dietary pattern and risk of treated diabetes mellitus in postmenopausal women: the Women's Health Initiative randomized controlled dietary modification trial." <u>Arch Intern Med</u> **168**(14): 1500-1511.

Tremblay, A., A. Nadeau, et al. (1995). "Hyperinsulinemia and regulation of energy balance." <u>Am J Clin Nutr</u> **61**(4): 827-830.

Ulrich-Lai, Y. M., M. M. Ostrander, et al. (2010). "HPA axis dampening by limited sucrose intake: Reward frequency vs. caloric consumption." <u>Physiol Behav</u>.

Veldhorst, M. A., M. S. Westerterp-Plantenga, et al. (2009). "Gluconeogenesis and energy expenditure after a high-protein, carbohydrate-free diet." <u>Am J Clin Nutr</u> **90**(3): 519-526.

Verhoeven, S., K. Vanschoonbeek, et al. (2009). "Long-term leucine supplementation does not increase muscle mass or strength in healthy elderly men." <u>Am J Clin Nutr</u> **89**(5): 1468-1475.

Vogt, M., A. Puntschart, et al. (2003). "Effects of dietary fat on muscle substrates, metabolism, and performance in athletes." <u>Med Sci Sports Exerc</u> **35**(6): 952-960.

Warburg, O., F. Wind, et al. (1927). "The Metabolism of Tumors in the Body." J Gen Physiol **8**(6): 519-530.

Weigle, D. S., P. A. Breen, et al. (2005). "A high-protein diet induces sustained reductions in appetite, ad libitum caloric intake, and body weight despite compensatory changes in diurnal plasma leptin and ghrelin concentrations." Am J Clin Nutr **82**(1): 41-48.

Willcox, B. J., T. A. Donlon, et al. (2008). "FOXO3A genotype is strongly associated with human longevity." Proc Natl Acad Sci U S A **105**(37): 13987-13992.

Woodhill, J. M., A. J. Palmer, et al. (1978). "Low fat, low cholesterol diet in secondary prevention of coronary heart disease." Adv Exp Med Biol **109**: 317-330.

Woodhouse, S. P., W. H. Sutherland, et al. (1984). "Physical training and fasting serum insulin levels in sedentary men." Clin Physiol **4**(6): 475-482.

Yancy, W. S., Jr., E. C. Westman, et al. (2010). "A randomized trial of a low-carbohydrate diet vs orlistat plus a low-fat diet for weight loss." Arch Intern Med **170**(2): 136-145.

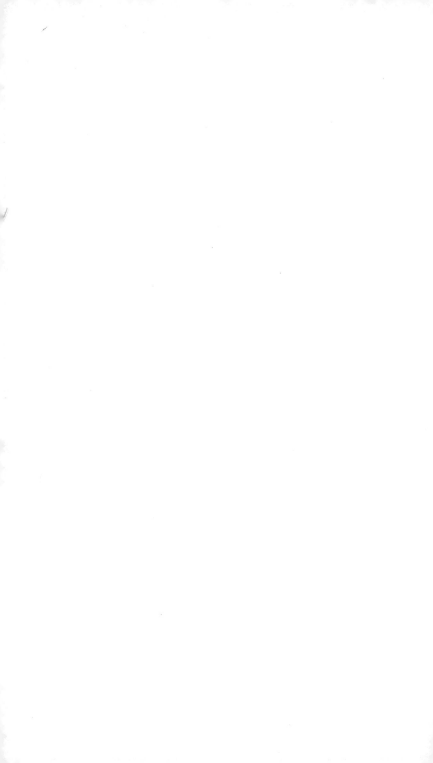